Teas for Life:

101 Herbal Teas
for
Greater Health

Teas for Life

101 Herbal Teas for Greater Health

Printed in the United States of America
ISBN: 978-0-9839155-7-7

Cover Design by: Diane Kidman

Published by: carp(e) libris press, LLC

Visit the Author Website at:
www.DianeKidman.com

Table of Contents

Introduction

If you've ever brewed a simple cup of tea, you've practiced herbalism. This most basic and ancient of acts has the power to deliver health and healing in a safer, more natural way to you and your family. And since it's so familiar to most of us, it's also a comfortable place to begin learning more about herbalism.

Teas for Life will help you break through the mystery around herbs and how to use them. Ever stand in the tea aisle with a box of dried marshmallow root in your hand and wonder what it's for? No, not S'mores. See, that's why you need this book. Keep it on you so next time you're out doing a bit of tea shopping, look that strange sounding herb up. Or if you're a gardener, find out if the lovely catmint plant is good for something other than pretty purple flowers and watching your cat get stoned. Maybe you recognize a few weedy items in your vegetable garden and feel a little bad about tossing them after the big yank. (I know about three of you must. I can't be the only one.) Find out if you can dry them and brew them.

Dandelion? It's tea. Ground ivy? You got it. Good stuff. By the time you go through this guide, you'll definitely have a shopping list or a gardening or weeding list made up so you can brew some health for that family of yours. Herbs, after all, are Nature's little health care plan. And Nature knows her stuff.

Warning: Nature will also tell you that it's important to view herbal teas with a healthy amount of respect. Although many of them are safe for everyday use, they all aren't. I've included warnings throughout the book, but the bottom line is that conflicting information abounds when we talk about herbs. Sometimes one herbalist will deem an herb perfectly safe, while another says it's not safe in certain instances. There have also been plenty of times when an herb considered safe by the vast majority of responsible herbalists will suddenly show up across the media with a strange side effect. But upon closer inspection of the facts, it turns out the "side effect" only occurs when you drink 27 gallons in one sitting while on a pharmaceutical known to cause loss of bladder control and off-key singing in middle aged men.

Then there are allergic reactions. I always say that for every substance on earth, there's at least one individual who's allergic. I don't like to plaster warnings all over the use of, say, chamomile when I know there's a good chance we could also find someone who breaks out into hives when they come into contact with corduroy. As Einstein would say, "It's all relative."

If you are on any prescription medications at all, it's important to make sure you can still take an herb. Check with your doctor. If your doctor doesn't know, ask the pharmacist or a health care professional versed in herbalism. Always exercise caution. Yes, herbs are usually safer than your average prescription drug. But there are ways to misuse herbs, too. Like stuffing them up your nose. That's never a good idea.

How to Use this Book

While a great many herbal references are organized alphabetically by the Latin names (which, incidentally, is the most reliable way to identify them), this book is first organized alphabetically by common name — or at least the most common name I know of. The common names are followed by the Latin names in parentheses. These are the names you should use when purchasing herbs. When you see a Latin name that includes "spp." that just means you can use any of the species in that particular genus. So, for instance, in the case of (*Pinus spp.*), this means any kind of pine tree will work and can be used in the same manner as the other kinds of pine trees. Except not Christmas trees. Don't make tea from Christmas trees. (Those are often treated or even spray painted.)

Uses: Each herb has a list of uses most commonly associated with that plant. This list isn't all-inclusive, by any means. So if you've had great success with an herb curing your nasty case of scurvy but I haven't mentioned that, it doesn't mean you've lost your mind or have experienced some strange power of suggestion. It does mean, however, that you should email me your scurvy story at themommyspot@gmail.com and let me know, because I find scurvy oddly fascinating and have never met anyone who had it.

Parts Used: This section lets you know what part of the herb has the medicinal qualities in question. If it says "whole herb," this means roots, leaves, stems, flowers, and all. If it says "whole above-ground plant," that's everything but the root. If you collect your own plants, that'll come in handy. If you purchase your herbs, this assures you're getting the part you want. Sometimes the root works totally different than the leaves, so if you're hoping to get the diuretic properties from the dandelion, you need to have the leaves on hand. Roots are for other good things.

Constituents: This is usually a long, complicated list of some of the known active parts and chemical makeup of the plants. I know it may make the plants look nightmarish. (Who knew chamomile contained alpha bisabolol, for heaven's sake?) But those are really the things that make these plants tick.

I say "known" active parts because we don't know everything in them. Part of the plants' mystique, if you will. And occasionally, you'll see a plant with no constituents listed at all. That doesn't mean there aren't any. It does mean that at the time of publication, I was unable to locate any reliable information. More is learned all the time, however, so if you're reading this and you're a weed scientist who sees my list isn't complete, all I can say is it was bound to happen at some point, smarty-pants.

If you need to discuss an herb with your healthcare professional and they aren't very familiar with herbs, the list of constituents may help them decide whether or not that plant is a good choice for you.

Dosage: Dosage recommendations can be found running all over the place for various medicinal plants, and that's usually okay. If you've been successful using a certain amount of tea that your herbalist told you was good to take but you see a discrepancy here, that's not always cause for concern. Just be sure that regardless of dosage, you keep in mind that moderation is always key.

Notes: I had to add the "Notes" section because I always have something to say about everything. Humor me.

Warnings: These are warnings to the best of my knowledge. I've compared numerous sources I trust, relied on personal experience, and taken as much care as I could to make sure the warnings are accurate. The bottom line is always to use caution and to consult with your doctor or a health care professional before making major changes. Do you need to call your doc and ask permission for a cup of chamomile tea before bed? Probably not. If you're taking 57 prescription meds, can you wash them all down with a cup of chamomile tea before bed? Probably not. But a bit of the old common sense and a call to the doctor when in doubt are always wise choices.

How to Brew Tea

If you're going to brew tea for medicinal purposes, you want to get the most out of the herb. While complicated instructions for brewing a "proper" herbal tea are often discussed in texts, and I often fuss over it plenty myself attempting to properly suspend the herb in water that's just the right temperature, the bottom line is, it's herbal tea. You can't mess it up that badly. So don't sweat it.

Some herbs do work better or different when prepared in cold water, what we call a "cold infusion." Others need hot water, or a "standard infusion." And yet others, such as the woody herbs, roots, and barks, release their best load of constituents when we do a "decoction," which simply means we simmer the plant material in the water instead of steeping it.

For the sake of this book, we'll be discussing how to make the tea by the cup. The vast majority of herbs will do just fine if you use 1 teaspoon of herb per an 8-ounce cup of water. While you don't actually need to drink the entire 8 ounces of tea in one sitting (as you'll see in the Dosage instructions of each herb), go ahead and make the full 8 ounces, anyway. The tea is good for up to 24 hours, so it's nice to prepare it and refrigerate any unused portions for a later dose, if needed.

Different herbalists prepare their herbs differently, some preferring to steep a certain plant while others insist decoction is better. Again, as your family's home herbalist, you've nothing to worry about there. This guide will tell you the preferred method in the Dosage section of each herb, so give that a try first. If you later decide that you like the way your pine needle tea comes out as a decoction as opposed to a standard infusion, go for it. Personally, I think that's kinda gross, but Bear Grylls does it all the time and he's still alive to talk about it. In the meantime, here's a quick guide to the different methods.

Equipment

We'll not discuss anything fancy here. The important thing is to keep it simple so you're not overcome with steps and new equipment. Sure, special teapots and fancy strainers do exist (and I'll admit to owning several impressive doohickeys myself), but they're not really needed. Just get a mug, something to boil water in, and a tea strainer of some sort. Tea balls are nice and inexpensive, and if you don't have one, it's the one thing I'd recommend you go out and get. But you don't even need one of those. You can just pour the water over the herb and strain it out with a teaspoon later. Just be forewarned: When you don't feel very well as it is, picking bits of herb out of a mug isn't very fun, nor is chewing twig remnants in between sips.

Standard Infusion

This is the most basic of methods, probably closest to what you already do. Simply bring 8 ounces of water to a boil, then pour the water over about a teaspoon of herb and cover. Allow it to sit for 20 to 30 minutes. This is much longer than for, say, a cup of black tea, but it's important to give the herb time to release all it has to give. Strain out the herb. If the water level is now less than 8 ounces, go ahead and add some fresh cold water to the cup to bring the water level back up.

Cold Infusion

In this instance, you'll need to make the tea the night before use. Place the herb inside your tea ball and run it under cold water just until moistened. You'll need to suspend the tea ball so it's at the top of the mug or container. If you have a tea ball with a chain, you can wrap the chain around the mug handle. Since the tea will need to be covered, I like to jerry-rig the tea ball under the lid or a small plate.

The herb needs to be suspended because the water molecules will be pulling the plant's constituents to the bottom of the container. When the molecules have pulled them down there, they float back up to the top to gather more. It makes a nice circulation of herb and water, brewing the tea over several hours.

In the morning, strain out the herb and add more cold water, if needed, to bring it back up to 8 ounces.

Strong (or Weak) Decoction

In a pan, combine 8 ounces of water with approximately one teaspoon of herb. Bring it to a slow boil and simmer for 10 minutes. Allow the tea to cool until warm, then strain out the herb. Add fresh water to bring the water level back to 8 ounces. For a weak decoction, just simmer for about 5 minutes.

In any of these cases, if you want to make more than 8 ounces, go right ahead. Perhaps you have quadruplets that have head colds, in which case you'll need a substantial amount of tea. While I sympathize, I'll hold back and let you do the calculations on herb to water.

Purchasing Herbs

There are a few dos and don'ts you should know when selecting the herbs you use as tea. The first no-no would be those colorful little boxes of herbal tea bags at the grocery store. While you may (if you're lucky) manage to get some decent herb, 12 teabags at $8 really equals 12 teaspoons of highly overpriced and possibly old herb. For that same $8, you might be able to wrangle yourself a whole pound (depending on the variety) of bulk herb, and you'll be able to see for yourself whether or not it's fresh before you've purchased it.

What's fresh dried herb? It should have color. Chamomile flowers should be white with yellow centers and smell kind of like apples. It shouldn't be a bag of stemmy green stuff with a smattering of petals. Rosemary should smell like rosemary — fresh, strong, invigorating. While it may take some experience to figure out what a particular herb should smell and look like, one thing is certain: If it's a bunch of dusty gray or brown leaf-type residue with little fragrance, it's probably no good.

If you're purchasing online, it's impossible to be able to sniff and see for yourself, but there are several reputable online herb stores. At the end of this book, I've put together an Herbal Shopping Guide with some links for you to check out.

Teas for Life lists the herbs in alphabetical order of their common names. Most plants have a handful of common names, so to avoid confusion, I've also included the Latin names. This will help you find exactly the right herb. Any herb store worth its salt will list their herbs using the proper Latin names.

Wildcrafting

If you're a more adventurous home herbalist, you can try your hand at wildcrafting. This is the process of pulling on the hiking boots, donning a silly floppy hat, and carting a banged-up duffle bag full of pruning shears, spades, blades, and bags for the collecting of herbs from the wild. It's herbalism at its finest, in my opinion, and it gives you a much deeper connection to your family medicine — somewhat like appreciating the food on your table more when you had to grow it yourself.

If you prefer to learn the art of wildcrafting, it's important above all else to know exactly what it is you're picking. No guessing or saying something looks close enough! While in America most plants aren't deadly, the few that are often resemble plants that are safe. So you must know what you're doing. For the amateur, get comfortable with just one or two plants at a time. Like dandelion. You may think I'm joking, but any herbalist worth her salt will have a store of dandelion. You'll need to know how to pick it, when to pick it, where to pick it, etc. While this is definitely a major endeavor, the rewards are great. My best suggestion is to seek out a qualified wildcrafter and either convince them to take you out herb gathering (a good bottle of red or some cold hard cash are good plies), so they can point things out to you and show you firsthand. Many herbalists offer day classes called "herb walks" in which they take groups of people out into the wild to learn about the proper identification and gathering techniques. They'll also let you know which plants to leave untouched, such as protected and poisonous species.

Growing Your Own Herbs

If you are fortunate enough to have a green thumb, you can grow just about anything you really need right in your own backyard. I always jest about being a terrible gardener, something that may sound strange coming from an herbalist (I'm much more comfortable with letting a plant do its own thing in the wild), but in truth, there are numerous herbs that thrive under neglect. Again, this is a case of gathering some good gardening books. And if you've no space for a garden, container gardening for both indoors and out can help you in growing your own medicine.

Now, let's get to those herbs. We'll start in the best place to start. The beginning.

A

Agrimony *(Agrimonia striata or eupatoria)*

Uses: Diarrhea in children, bedwetting. Appendicitis. Indigestion. Good for acute cystitis and/or urethritis with cloudy, smelly urine and incontinence, severe pain. Left-over pain after food poisoning. Also relieves heavy uterine feeling during menses, menstrual pain and cramping. Hypermetabolic or overactive liver from things such as drug excess or chemotherapy. Cirrhosis, jaundice, hepatitis. Bronchitis, asthma, whooping cough. Also good for the flu when intermittent chills are present, as well as achy joints. Stressed out people who tend to hide it all away often benefit from agrimony. Relieves tension headaches, allergic welts brought on by stress. Good after being in too much sun.

Parts Used: Herb

Constituents: Tannins, flavonoids, coumarins, polysaccharides, trace amounts of minerals and glycosidal bitters.

Dosage: Standard infusion, 2 to 4 ounces as needed.

Notes: Agrimony is a safe herb that can be used regularly. It's enjoyed a long history of herbalism use and has been relied upon for some of the above ailments for hundreds of years, and there is lots of good folklore surrounding it. It was once said that if you kept agrimony under your pillow, there'd be no waking up until the herb was removed. Perhaps that was Rip Van Wikle's problem. I knew all he needed was a good herbalist.

Warnings: None known.

Alchemilla, Lady's Mantle (*Alchemilla vulgaris*)

Uses: For women, this is especially good for fibroids and endometriosis and can bring relief (but won't cure) profuse bleeding during menses. Vaginitis, yeast infection, leucorrhea. Uterine or bladder atony, prolapse. Nervousness, mood swings. Headaches and cramps associated with PMS. Strengthening to the heart and atria; also strengthens weak muscles, abdominal walls, the pelvic floor and the uterus. Diarrhea. Bleeding disorders. Also good for feverish children with sore throats and upper respiratory distress.

Parts Used: Whole budding plant

Constituents: Tannins, trace amounts of salicylic acid.

Dosage: Two teaspoons per cup of water. Standard infusion as needed.

Notes: Lady's mantle was one of the most popular medicinal herbs of the Middle Ages. Renaissance doctors relied on it heavily for women's issues, and they had it right because many women still keep it within reach.

Warnings: None known.

Alfalfa (*Medicago sativa*)

Uses: Improves a poor appetite in those feeling weak and nervous, in particularly when recovering from surgery or a major illness or those suffering from malnutrition. It's a highly nutritive herb that is rich in minerals, thus making it an excellent spring tonic. Boosts lactation quality and quantity. Helps prevent heart disease and lowers high blood pressure; thins the blood. Good for diverticulitis, sluggish bowels, and constipation. Upper respiratory tract support; hay fever and allergies, nosebleeds. Supports anemic types and is good for convalescing individuals. Relieves boils, itchy and irritable skin, rashes. Especially nice for arthritis and gout.

Parts Used: Flowering plant

Constituents: Calcium, folic acid, vitamin K.

Dosage: Standard infusion as needed.

Notes: Alfalfa isn't just a funny little kid with a cow lick. It's also one of the most ancient crops in humanity. It improves your calcium absorption and gives you a nutritive boost. And cows love it, too.

Warnings: Mild side effects such as gas, bloating, and/or diarrhea sometimes occur. Long-term usage can result in a resurgence of SLE (systemic lupus erythematosus) in those who currently have inactive lupus. May be inappropriate for pregnant women, or for men and women with infertility problems.

American Saffron (*Carthamus tinctorius*)

Uses: Helpful in cases of measles and other eruptive skin issues such as chicken pox; fine for children. An old folk remedy for smallpox. Boils and hives. Relieves suppressed menses due to a recent viral infection. Also relieves menstrual pain. Laxative and diuretic. Softens hardened phlegm due to asthma, tuberculosis, bronchitis, and general cough. Stimulates a weak appetite. Good for diverticulitis and stomach ulcers. Diarrhea and constipation.

Parts Used: Flowers

Constituents: Flavonoid glycosides.

Dosage: Standard infusion, 4 to 8 ounces up to 3 times daily.

Notes: Okay, so it's really safflower. But the alternate name of American saffron sounds much more elegant, don't you think? While I doubt they called it American saffron, the ancient Egyptians liked using it. One of the oldest crop plants known, even King Tut was buried with garlands of it. If it's fit for a king, my friend, it is definitely fit for you.

Warnings: None known.

American Sarsaparilla (*Aralia nudicaulis*)

Uses: An aromatic plant that works well as an expectorant and for cold congestion within the lungs, as well as other lung ailments; mild stimulant. Builds up the stressed out individual. Rheumatism, stomach aches. Adrenal insufficiency. Hyperlipidemia.

Parts Used: Root is most common; good to use whole plant when available.

Constituents: Steroids, sarsasapogenin, smilagenin, sitosterol, stigmasterol, pollinastrenol, glycosides, saponins, sarsasaponin parillin, smilasaponin, smilacin, sarsaparilloside, sitosterol glucoside.

Dosage: Cold infusion, 2 to 4 ounces up to 3 times daily.

Notes: American sarsaparilla is considered an adaptogen, which means it helps the body adapt when under stress. It's a good wintertime tonic for people who live in colder regions and are more susceptible to lung issues. And, yes, cowboys used to drink a "sody pop" made out of it.

Warnings: None known.

Angelica (*Angelica archangelica*)

Uses: Expectorant action makes this a nice choice for coughs due to cold, flu, pleurisy, and bronchitis, especially when paired with a fever. Flatulence, intestinal colic relief. Appetite stimulant sometimes used to treat anorexia nervosa. Cystitis. Rheumatism.

Parts Used: Root, leaf

Constituents: Volatile oils, a- and B-phellandrene, a-pinene, a-thujene, limonene, B-caryophyllene, linalool, borneol, acetaldehyde, macrocyclic lactones, phthalates, furanocoumarin glycosides, sugars, plant acids, flavonoids, sterols.

Dosage: Strong decoction, 1 to 2 ounces up to 4 times daily.

Notes: Angelica root was used to create a popular candy once upon a time. While you'll be hard pressed to find the candy form anymore, it's still one of the ingredients in gin. And, no, drinking gin won't relieve your rheumatism, despite what Grandma tried to tell you.

Warnings: May cause photosensitivity, so avoid prolonged exposure to the sun and UV rays while taking it. Consult with your health care professional before taking angelica when using anticoagulant medications.

Aniseed (*Pimpinella anisum*)

Uses: Asthma, bronchitis, whooping cough, coughing in general. Mild lung expectorant and stimulant; especially nice for children. Aids in digestion. Relief from griping pains, indigestion, and intestinal colic. Can stimulate sweating, so in the case of fever, drink as hot as can be tolerated.

Parts Used: Seeds

Constituents: Volatile oil, mostly trans-anethole, dianethole, and photoanethole; coumarins; flavonoids; phenylpropanoids; lipids; fatty acids; sterols; proteins; carbohydrates.

Dosage: Steep a pinch of seeds in a standard infusion; drink as needed.

Notes: This is a nice herb for children. It's pleasant tasting, naturally sweet, and mild.

Warnings: None known.

Arbor Vitae (*Thuja occidentalis*)

Uses: This is a highly antifungal herb which works very well for things such as Candida, jock itch, athlete's foot, ringworm, and urinary tract infections. Immunostimulant; slows bacterial growth. Chronic cystitis or urethritis with prostatitis. Good for older men who have enlarged prostates and experience incontinence or insufficient bladder control. Acute vulvitis with burning irritation. Amoebic dysentery, giardia.

Parts Used: Herb

Constituents: Volatile oil including thujone, flavonoid glycosides, mucilage, tannins.

Dosage: Cold infusion, 2 to 3 ounces up to 3 times daily.

Notes: For things such as athlete's foot and ringworm, apply it topically.

Warnings: Not to be used internally during pregnancy.

Artichoke *(Cynara scolymus)*

Uses: Supports healthy liver function. Helps prevent gall stones. Dyspepsia, irritable bowel syndrome, Crohn's disease, constipation. Also good for cardiovascular health. Helps in the digestion of fats and the metabolizing of sugar. Decreases appetite. Diuretic.

Parts Used: Flowering herb

Constituents: Cynarine, sesquiterpene lactones, inulin, flavonoids, polyphenols, caffeic acids, tannins, zinc, nickel, cobalt, manganese, selenium, enzymes.

Dosage: Standard infusion, 2 to 4 ounces up to 3 times daily. Drink before meals.

Notes: Artichokes used to be totally inaccessible unless you were rich. If you've ever wondered why the artichoke shows up in interior design schemes or articles of antiquity, now you know. It was a status symbol. Which is why I serve the dip at parties.

Warnings: Some people experience contact dermatitis by touching the fresh leaf. Other people are just jealous because I make a better dip.

Astragalus (*Astragalus membranaceus*)

Uses: An excellent immunostimulant, it strengthens several immune system functions. Also protects the liver from damage. Cystitis or urethritis with systemic infections and/or fever. Septic diarrhea. Septicemia.

Parts Used: Root

Constituents: Triterpenoid saponin glycosides, flavonoid glycosides and aglycones, cycloastragenol, high-molecular-weight polysaccharides.

Dosage: Cold infusion, 2 to 3 ounces up to 3 times daily.

Notes: Astragalus is being studied due to its impressive knack for stimulating the immune system. According to a study in the *Journal of Immunology* (Nov. 2008), the root has the ability to slow the aging process in immune cells. One constituent of the plant, cycloastragenol, has researchers wondering if it can end the HIV virus, but only time will tell.

Warnings: If taking immunosuppressive drugs, please consult with your physician before using.

B

Barberry (*Berberis vulgaris*)

Uses: Promotes the flow of bile and corrects liver function. Remedy for gallstones and gallbladder inflammation. Mild laxative. Relieves biliousness due to overeating or drug excesses. Dyspepsia after fatty foods. Vomiting during pregnancy. Cleanses the system in the weak or debilitated individual. Reduces enlarged spleens. Eczema. Acute psoriasis. Migraines that hurt even more when moving. Sore, burning eyes; dry, itching eyes. Antimalarial.

Parts Used: Root or stem bark

Constituents: Isoquinoline alkaloids, chelidonic acid, resin, tannins.

Dosage: Cold infusion, 1 to 3 ounces up to 3 times daily.

Notes: Some herbalists stick to the idea that barberry is not for pregnant women, while others recommend it to

33

reduce vomiting. It is an extremely bitter herb, which makes it difficult to overdo the tea — you just wouldn't want to drink that much of it. Still, if you're pregnant and want to take barberry, discuss it with your doctor or midwife first.

Warnings: If pregnant, consult your health care professional before use.

Betony *(Pedicularis spp.)*

Uses: Good sedative for hyperactive kids and adults. Relaxing to the skeletal muscles; relieves muscle spasms and lessens muscular pain, especially in children. Insomnia caused by overexcitement. Good for gastrointestinal irritability, chronic rheumatism, strokes, ischemic headaches, sciatica.

Parts Used: Herb in flower or bud

Constituents: Iridoid and phenylpropanoid glycosides; flavonoids.

Dosage: Standard infusion, 4 to 8 ounces up to 4 times daily.

Notes: If you have the uncomfortable issue of falling asleep and jerking yourself awake, try mixing betony with passionflower. Just don't overdo the betony, though. It's so relaxing it can make you kinda drooly.

Warnings: This is a pretty safe herb, but for some people it really affects them and makes them a bit too relaxed. So try it in a smaller dose first until you know how it will affect you.

Birch (*Betula alba*)

Uses: Dry coughing due to being pent up indoors with forced air heat, etc; tea of the leaves is best in this instance. Cystitis, bladder, and other urinary tract infections. Diarrhea, cholera, and dysentery. Kidney stones. Gout, rheumatism, mild arthritis pain. Stiff knees. Overworked muscles, tendons, and joints. Insomnia. Arteriosclerosis. Prolonged menses. Slow recovery after childbirth. For eczema, psoriasis, boils, abscesses, and acne, use externally. Also good for burns, wounds, cuts, etc., when used externally.

Parts Used: Bark

Constituents: Hyperoside, quercetin, flavonoids.

Dosage: Strong decoction, 1 to 2 ounces up to 4 times daily.

Notes: Birch tea also makes an excellent hair rinse, bringing it health and shine while improving the overall quality.

Warnings: None known.

Black Cohosh (*Cimicifuga racemosa*)

Uses: Chronic bronchitis, asthma, pneumonia. Whooping cough in children. Mumps with muscular aching. Rheumatoid ache in orbits of the eyes, ophthalmalgia. Eyestrain with a bruised sensation and headache. Ear pain caused by exposure to cold; rheumatic pain in inner ear. Flu with malaise and achiness. Sore bronchi. Delirium tremens, epilepsy, petit mal. Insomnia with muscle pain. Anorexia nervosa. Sprains with dull aches. Tendonitis. Cervical and ovarian neuralgia. Periodic convulsions brought on by uterine disorders. Used in Native American medicine for rheumatism and for women's issues, such as PMS, menopause, and uterine pains. Menopause with uterine pain brought on by any movement or jostling. Stress-related symptoms of menopause and premenopause. Mittelschmerz (that pinchy pain that happens about two weeks before menses, caused by the release of the egg from the ovary) with diarrhea or cramping of the colon. Dull, aching uterus. Chronic vaginitis. Good for helping through the menopause process while stimulating circulation and sedating the central nervous system.

Parts Used: Roots and rhizome are most popular in commerce, but foliage works just as well.

Constituents: Triterpene glycosides, cimifugoside, isoflavones, and aromatic acids.

Dosage: 1 heaping tsp. to a cup of water. Standard decoction, 1 to 4 times daily.

Notes: Black Cohosh is an expert at balancing the hormone levels in both men and women. In women, it's often used instead of estrogen replacement therapy (ERT). Unlike ERT, it may actually prevent tumor growth in breast cancer, much the opposite of ERT which is believed to speed up breast cancer tumor growth.

Warnings: Moderate or large doses may cause a sense of unpleasantness or cramping. Not for use during early pregnancy. Any use during pregnancy at all should be under the direction of a trained professional.

Blackberry (*Rubus fruticosus*)

Uses: Diarrhea, especially in children. Sore throat, cough, whooping cough with spasmodic coughing fits. Anemia, dropsy. Digestive issues that are paired with headaches and sensations of sluggishness. Eczema. Hemorrhoids, varicose veins, ulcers. For heavy menses with dull aching in the abdomen, use the whole herb. Also good during late pregnancy to aid in birthing.

Parts Used: Root and/or root bark and/or leaf, although root is the more traditional and often believed to be more effective.

Constituents: Tannins, gallic acid, saponins.

Dosage: Strong decoction, 2 - 4 ounces up to 4 times daily.

Notes: In the end, all the Rubus plants are interchangeable. So if you don't have access to blackberry but raspberry leaf is more easy for you to come by, use that one instead.

Warnings: An excellent tonic for pregnancy; however, it should only be used during the last trimester and kept at reasonable amounts. One or two cups of tea a day is usually sufficient.

Blue Cohosh (*Caulophyllum thalictroides*)

Uses: Very good at toning the uterine muscles. Amenorrhea in young women; painful menstruation or a painful uterus; ovarian irritation. General PMS symptoms such as irritation, painful breasts, etc. Good for the relief of a heavy, sore feeling within the uterus accompanied by pain in the legs. Endometriosis, vaginitis, ovaritis, urethritis, cervicitis. Menopausal pains which refer down into the legs; also with pain in ovaries, uterus, sacrum, bladder, and having a sense of general confusion and nervousness. Insomnia. Spasmodic muscle pain such as with rheumatism. Asthma, bronchitis, whooping cough. Arthritis pain, especially that which occurs in smaller joints like fingers and toes. Sometimes used in cases of epilepsy, as it is a cerebrospinal trophorestorative.

Parts Used: Rhizome

Constituents: Methylcytisine, caulophyllosaponin, caulosaponin.

Dosage: Standard decoction; 1 heaping teaspoon decocted in 8 ounces of water, 1 to 4 times a day.

Notes: If you gather your own plants for medicinal use, make sure you dry the roots of the blue cohosh thoroughly. There are a few plants out there, such as this one, which are susceptible to molding and fermentation when used fresh. Occasionally, someone will be sensitive to these molds, so dry the root completely before use.

Warnings: Some women experience mid-cycle spotting or cramping while using this herb. Not for use within the first seven months of pregnancy. Blue cohosh can stress an unborn baby's heart, so if using within the last two months of pregnancy, it should be done with great care and under the supervision of a health professional who is knowledgeable on the use of the herb. Overdose may cause nausea, vomiting, dilated pupils, headache, thirst, incoordination. Not for those with angina or cardiac weaknesses.

Blueberry (*Vaccinium spp.*)

Uses: In juvenile onset insulin-dependent diabetes, it can lessen insulin use. Stabilizes blood sugar levels. An excellent tea for hypoglycemics, as it provides a quick source of blood sugar without causing a sudden spike and drop of sugar levels. Also a good choice for those with hyperinsulinism, aiding in keeping regular blood sugar levels. Tired eyes from computer use. Stimulates urine. Strengthens heartbeat. Relief of swollen prostate. Unlike the sweet fruits, blueberry leaves are highly astringent and antiseptic.

Parts Used: Leaves

Constituents: Polyphenols, caffeoyl quinic acids, flavonol glycosides, flavan-3-ols, proanthocyanidins., vaccinin A.

Dosage: Standard infusion, 3 to 4 ounces up to 3 times daily. Freshly dried leaves preferred.

Notes: In my neck of the woods, huckleberries abound. The leaves of the huckleberry can be used in the same way as the blueberry leaves. If you have your own bushes, make sure you use only leaves that have not been sprayed or treated, and that you can safely make a positive identification.

Warnings: None known.

Boneset (*Eupatorium perfoliatum*)

Uses: Good for head colds and viral infections that are accompanied by moist fevers and aches. Acute bronchitis, hot and dry, with weakness in muscles; acute bronchial pneumonia; pleurisy. Achy flu with general malaise. Immune stimulant, fever reducer, pain reducer, expectorant. Helpful with weak and unproductive coughs. Expels metabolic waste. Also good for chicken pox, measles, German measles, and any virus that includes skin eruptions, as it brings on the eruptions more quickly, reducing the risk of damage. As the name suggests, it is helpful to the bones. It brings pain relief to aching bones and muscles, helps repair damage to connective tissue and to broken bones, recalcifies the bones, and rebuilds the myelin sheaths in cases of multiple sclerosis.

Parts Used: Flowering herb

Constituents: Sesquiterpene lactones, immunostimulatory polysaccharides, flavonoids, diterpenes, sterols, volatile oil.

Dosage: As a tonic, cold infusion; to induce sweating, standard infusion. Both forms, 2 to 6 ounces up to 3 times a day.

Notes: During the 1918 - 1919 flu epidemic, boneset was the herb of choice and was touted as a miracle due to its success. I always have some in the house. If it's effective enough for a major flu epidemic, it's effective enough for my little family!

Warnings: Some people can experience contact dermatitis from touching the herb in its fresh form.

Bugleweed (*Lycopus americanus*)

Uses: Hyperthyroidism, hyperadrenalism; exophthalmic goiter (bulging of the eye) from long-term hyperthyroidism. Chronic nosebleed. Chronic bronchitis; the coughing up of blood. Mild bleeding in the urinary tract, intestines, stomach, uterus, or lungs. Over-rapid GI transit time. Anxiety, tachycardia with excitement. Palpitations after an infection that included a fever. Irregular heartbeat. Insomnia. Sedative to the circulatory system and heart; nervous system sedative. Asthma associated with hyperthyroidism. Scarlet fever, or for those who have had scarlet fever and haven't felt right since. Diarrhea, dysentery.

Parts Used: Herb

Constituents: Phenolic acid derivatives, pimaric acid methyl ester.

Dosage: Standard infusion of the recently dried plant, 2 to 3 ounces up to 3 times daily. (While the infusion is helpful, many of the constituents can be damaged with hot water. You may consider taking this one as a tincture instead.)

Notes: Bugleweed reduces the body's output of thyroid-stimulating hormone, or TSH. People with hyperthyroidism who feel especially wound up and can't sleep may find this to be their herb.

Warnings: Not for use in cases of enlarged thyroid or hypothyroid (underactive thyroid). If using thyroid medications, consult your physician before use. If pregnant, consult your physician or midwife. Do not use if nursing. Those with severe coronary artery disease should not use the herb.

Burdock (*Arctium minus*)

Uses: Chronic herpes; chronic canker sores. Good for long-term use as a chronic acne, eczema, or psoriasis treatment. Helps heal skin ulcers, hives, acne boils, sebaceous cysts. Lowers lipids in arteriosclerosis. For blood serum levels, it works on cholesterol elevations, hyperlipidemia, uric acid elevation, and acidosis. Eliminates toxins in the bloodstream and purifies lymph. Helps eliminate metabolic waste, especially to skin, kidneys, and mucous membranes. Hepatitis, kidney stones. Pulls gut toxins out of the body via water

45

soluble fibers. Supports beneficial flora in the gut, hence it's a great choice for Candida and colitis. Aids in allergies, sinusitis, bronchitis, and other respiratory conditions that include dry mucosa. Gout with excess uric acid production. Supports a compromised or weak immune system. Sciatica which becomes intolerable at night. Carpal tunnel syndrome. Profuse sweating under the arms. Regulates menstrual cycle during menopause. Mastitis remedy.

Parts Used: Root

Constituents: Antitumor lignins, artiin, arctigenin, fatty oils. Polysaccharides, volatile oils, inulin, tannins, mucilage, calcium, phosphorus, sodium, iron, thiamin, riboflavin, niacin, ascorbic acid, quercetin, nobiletin, tangeretin, natural flavones including the isoflavones genistein and biochanin A.

Dosage: Cold infusion, 2 to 4 ounces up to 3 times daily.

Notes: Most well known for its sticky burs that cling to anyone and anything, burdock was first cultivated by the Japanese thousands of years ago. Originally grown as food, it "escaped" as so many plants now considered weeds once did. It's still edible, though, and very popular in Japan. You can purchase burdock in Asian food stores here in the U.S., or you can brave the wild burs and gather it yourself.

Warnings: Although burdock root is even safe as a food, occasionally someone with an allergy to Asteraceae plants may find they can't tolerate it. There is a slight chance you may experience skin outbreaks when using burdock; this may be due to burdock's cleansing effect on the system.

C

Calamus, Sweet Flag (*Acorus calamus*)

Uses: A nice relaxing herb that's cooling to the stomach. A good antispasmodic, hence good for lower intestinal cramps, menstrual cramps, diarrhea, and dysentery. Flatulent or gastric colic. Relieves projective vomiting. Also helps cramping of bile ducts, gall bladder, ureters. Eases painful first days of menses. Helps some women with endometriosis. In cases of anorexia nervosa or anorexia as a result of chemotherapy, calamus can make food appear less vile. Also for nervousness, head injury, senility. Bronchitis, asthma.

Parts Used: Leaves. (Rhizome if using as a tincture, which is more effective than the tea.)

Constituents: Bitters, asarone, calamene, eugenol.

Dosage: Standard infusion, 2 to 4 ounces up to 4 times daily.

Notes: Acorus calamus was brought to America from Europe and has a vanilla-like flavor which was sometimes used by settlers as a vanilla extract. Native American tribes used to carry the variety (Americanus calamus), or American calamus, with them on long journeys. It has the unique effect of offering a quickness of perception the ancient peoples found helpful during long and arduous travel. Personally, I'd like some just to get to the grocery store and back.

Warnings: Certain genotypes of calamus contain carcinogens, in particular the European varieties. Care should be taken.

Calendula *(Calendula officinalis)*

Uses: Herpes simplex with secondary bacterial infection. Can be used as an external rinse for vaginal warts. Menopausal fibroids, leucorrhea. Varicose veins, hemorrhoids. Swollen glands. Lingering infections, both internal and external. Soothes digestive mucosa. Bronchitis and asthma associated with old infections. Use as a mouth rinse for gum disease or mouth ulcers. Upset stomach, vomiting, ulcers, diarrhea. Skin ulcers, abscesses, puss-filled infections, ulcerations, etc., if used externally. It decreases the possibility of scarring and promotes healing. Anti-inflammatory. Antibacterial and antiviral when used topically. Also as a topical use, it's good for abrasions, burns, cuts, stings, bruises, blisters, measles, chicken pox, frostbite, acne. Relieves pain in external applications.

Parts Used: Flowers

Constituents: Flavonoids, polysaccharides, bitters, resins, saponins, carotenes, xanthophylls, tannins, volatile oils, and minerals (including iodine).

Dosage: Standard infusion, 2 to 3 Tbs. steeped in 8 oz. of water. Drink as needed.

Notes: Traditionally, calendula is considered a winter tonic in Europe, taken throughout the season to help with immunity against all those nasty cold weather ailments. When purchasing calendula, the more orange the flower, the fresher it is. As dried calendula ages, it turns yellow. Always look for the orange flowers.

Warnings: Not to be used during pregnancy, as it can have abortifacient effects.

California Poppy (*Eschscholzia californica*)

Uses: Antispasmodic, anti-anxiety. Good for restlessness and insomnia for adults or children. Useful both in cases of sleep that's not deep and sleep that's too deep. For painful urination with little results. Colic in children. Bedwetting in children, especially when caused by nervousness. Headache, toothache, general neuropathies. Relieves tinnitus caused by exposure to loud noise, such as the morning after a rock concert.

Parts Used: Flowering plant

Constituents: Californidine, escholidine, protopine, N-methyllaurotanin, allocryptopine, sanguinarine.

Dosage: Standard infusion, 2 to 4 ounces up to 3 times daily.

Notes: The sedative alkaloids in California poppy are similar to those in the opium poppy plant, but without all the hassle of being addictive, illegal, depressing, narcotic, etc. The

California poppy is a safe plant, even for children. And no one will go to jail for drinking the tea.

Warnings: Before using during pregnancy, consult your physician or midwife. Do not use if taking an MAO inhibitor.

Canadian Fleabane (*Conyza canadensis*, formerly called *Erigeron canadensis*)

Uses: A good astringent herb that is abundant in the wild. Bleeding hemorrhoids, especially those that are irritating for days but don't bleed a lot; also good for diverticulitis under similar conditions. Especially good for irritable bowel syndrome (IBS) and ulcerative colitis with occasional bleeding. Diarrhea in general. Bleeding ulcers. Post-partum hemorrhage. Conjunctivitis. Chronic cough with profuse discharge, chronic bronchitis, tuberculosis. Hay fever and allergies with profuse bronchial secretions. Also relieves congestion due to inflammation. Suppressed or painful menses. Profuse urination. Chronic urethritis, cystitis. Rheumatism and gout. Profuse sweating.

Parts Used: Flowering herb, recently dried (within a year or two)

Constituents: Limonene, dipentene, proprionic acid, gallic acid, terpineol, methyl caprate derivatives.

Dosage: Standard infusion, 2 to 4 ounces up to 4 times daily.

Notes: While this plant is not easily found in commerce, it is definitely worth mentioning here, as it is possibly the best herbal remedy for ulcerative colitis and IBS. It is extremely common throughout North America, Mexico, and Europe, and is sprinkled elsewhere in the world. For distribution maps to see if it grows near you, along with some good images, check www.eol.org.

Warnings: Some people who have allergies to plants in the Asteraceae family may be allergic to Canadian fleabane.

Caraway (*Carum carvi*)

Uses: Aids in digestion. Good for flatulent colic in adults and in infants. Upset stomachs with belching and gas. Ironically, it's also good as an appetite stimulant.

Parts Used: Seed

Constituents: Protein, carbohydrate, flavonoids, a fixed oil, and an essential oil containing carvone and limonene.

Dosage: Standard infusion of 1 tsp. crushed seeds to 8 oz. of boiling water, as needed.

Notes: This is a simple remedy with a few basic functions, but it serves those functions very well indeed. It's safe for all ages and is a great addition to anyone's home herbal collection. It's antimicrobial, which is why it solves stomach issues well. It's also highly antifungal.

Warnings: None known.

Catclaw Acacia (*Acacia greggii*)

Uses: Laryngitis and acute pharyngitis as a gargle. Acute gastritis. Can be used externally for "pink eye" or conjunctivitis. Excellent remedy for diarrhea and dysentery. Highly astringent, it's good to stop the bleeding on cuts, scrapes, abrasions, etc., when applied topically. Tea of the flowers and leaves works well to stop nausea and vomiting, and it can provide hangover relief. Works as a sedative.

Parts Used: Pods and/or leaves

Constituents: Benzyl alcohol, butyric acid, coumarin, cresol, 7',3',4'-trihydroxyflavan-3, 4-diol, leucoanthocyanidin, N-methyl-B-phenethylamine, N-methylpentathylamine, N-methyltyramine, tyramine, gum, anisaldehyde, benzoic acid.

Dosage: Standard infusion, 2 to 4 ounces up to 5 times daily.

Notes: Not to be confused with the herb cat's claw (*Uncaria tomentosa*). Catclaw acacia is usually found in the Southwest U.S. and is also nicknamed "wait-a-minute." If you manage to run into this tree, you'll definitely have to tell everyone else to wait a minute as you carefully extricate yourself from its hooked thorns.

Warnings: None known.

Catmint *(Nepeta cataria)*

Uses: Nervous indigestion with agitation. Nausea, vomiting, stomachache, cramps in infants, children, and adults. Colic in infants that includes flatulence, crying, hysteria, great agitation. Fever or teething in infants and children. Headache with moist skin in children. Motion sickness. Cold or flu with a fever; it's able to produce sweating without first raising internal temperature, making it a safe choice for all ages. Headaches brought on by nerves. Mild sedative, antispasmodic. Menstrual discomfort with agitation (be sure to drink hot.) A great herb for insomnia. A good herb for worriers. Anxiety attack relief. Good for someone who's had too much coffee and needs to settle down. When used externally, it relieves skin irritations such as hives, scarlatina, measles, etc. Relaxes the brain, quiets the temper.

Parts Used: Flowering herb

Constituents: Contains an essential oil made up of carvacrol, nepetol, thymol, and nepetalactone; iridoids; tannins.

Dosage: Standard infusion of ¼ to 1 tsp., as needed.

Notes: This is a good herb for infants and small children. Please refer to Clark's Rule at the end of this book to figure proper dosage for your child or infant. Nursing mothers may consider taking the herb themselves, thus passing it to the infant through the breast milk. It'll settle the colic and sweeten the milk, not to mention relax a frazzled new mom.

Catmint is also my preferred choice for insomnia. It's mild enough that you don't feel drugged up and trippy if, instead of getting to go to bed after taking it, you have to sit up with a sick child. But it works. No funny dreams, no waking up in the morning forgetting your name. Just a good, safe sleep.

Warnings: Not to be used by pregnant women due to abortifacient effects.

Celery Seed *(Apium graveolens)*

Uses: A nerve tonic and sedative, it's great for anxiety, panic attacks, nervous breakdowns, insomnia. Also a good choice for arthritis, rheumatism, gout, indigestion, flatulence, kidney stones, and bladder stones. Helpful in rheumatoid arthritis that brings on a depression. Helps urinary tract inflammation and infection. Throbbing headaches. Neuralgia. Cold, flu, asthma, bronchitis, emphysema. Lack of appetite. Jaundice. Hypertension. Water retention. Amenorrhea. PMS. Irritated prostate.

Parts Used: Seed

Constituents: Volatile oil, limonene, selenine, a-eudesmol and b-eudesmol, santalol, phthalides, furanocoumarins, flavonoids.

Dosage: Simple infusion of ½ to 1 tsp. seeds in 8 oz. hot water. Take as needed.

Notes: I really like celery seed. While the tea is a bit reminiscent of drinking weak soup, the results are very nice indeed. It offers relaxation that feels like you're floating over

59

your problems instead of being smack in the middle of them. It's safe for regular use, so if you or someone you know suffers from panic attacks or anxiety, this is an excellent herb to keep around. Works well as a tincture, too.

Warnings: Use moderately in pregnancy or with kidney disorders only after you check with your health care professional. Some herbalists claim celery seed has abortifacient results when taken in large quantities.

Chamomile (*Matricaria spp.*)

Uses: A highly useful herb that aids in any discomfort that includes stomachache and sleeplessness. Insomnia and nightmares. Indigestion and epigastric fullness, especially with food fermentation. Nervous indigestion. Nausea, both general and morning sickness. Ulcers. Colic or fever in infants with crying and agitation. Infant teething. Children in their "terrible twos" who have been amped up a bit too long and just need to take things down a notch. Headache and/or vomiting in children; also diarrhea. Eczema; apply topically. Bath for arthritis or gout relief. Achy joints due to shifts in the weather. Cold and flu relief, as well as fever reducer, for all ages. PMS, menstrual cramping with low flow. Nervousness in pregnancy. Bedwetting caused by a bladder infection. Irritable nervousness at any age. Good as an eyewash for conjunctivitis or irritated eyes. The warm tea can also be used to relieve ear pain when used as ear drops. Anti-inflammatory, both internal and external.

Parts Used: Flowers

Constituents: Sesquiterpenes, sesquiterpene lactones, flavonoid glycosides, apigenin, luteolin, quercetin, isorhamnetin.

Dosage: Standard or cold infusion, 2 to 6 ounces up to 4 times daily.

Notes: Don't underestimate the powers of chamomile. It shouldn't be viewed as just a tea for little old ladies who need a "sleepytime" aid. Yes, it's mild enough for babies and small children, but as you can see, the list of uses is seemingly endless. And while most herbal teas lose much of their efficacy by sitting on the back of a store shelf in old teabags, chamomile still retains a surprising amount of usefulness, even when it's nothing more than herb dust and stems. Of course, if

61

you really want its full benefit, get it freshly dried or grow it yourself. It's an easy garden plant, and the difference in taste, smell, and potency is significant.

Warnings: None known

Chicory (*Cichorium intybus*)

Uses: Headachy feverishness. Bronchitis, lung congestion, especially good for children. Stomach upset from food; crampy, sense of indigestion. Anemia, atrophy, malnourishment. Sick, weak individuals with weak stomachs. Arthritis, gout. Pimples, rashes, skin irritations. Mastitis.

Parts Used: Root

Constituents: Inulin (not to be confused with insulin), caffeoylquinic acids.

Dosage: Strong decoction, 3 to 6 ounces up to 4 times daily.

Notes: Chicory isn't just a good tea. It's a lovely coffee substitute! Many coffee substitute blends contain chicory root, and it's a traditional beverage in Europe. For this use, the roots are slow roasted, then ground and brewed just like coffee. I've roasted my own, and I love the smell. It's amazing how similar it is to the smell of roasting coffee beans.

Warnings: None known.

Chickweed (*Stellaria media*)

Uses: A good diuretic to be used for premenstrual relief. Also relieves water retention in people with sodium retention or rheumatism. Nice used topically for hemorrhoids, cuts and abrasions, burns, skin eruptions, eczema, psoriasis, and the like.

Parts Used: Whole above-ground herb

Constituents: Saponin glycosides, coumarins and hydroxycoumarins, flavonoids, carboxylic acids, triterpenoids, vitamin C.

Dosage: Standard infusion, 4 to 8 ounces up to 4 times daily.

Notes: This is a common yard "weed" and is best used in its fresh state. You can prepare it as a tea, or even juice it if you have a juicer. But make sure that if you gather it yourself, you are very comfortable with its identification. Also make sure you're not picking herb that has been sprayed with pesticides, fertilizers, etc.

Warnings: None known.

Cinnamon (*Cinnamomum spp.*)

Uses: Passive post-partum hemorrhage due to a lack of contractions. Also good for excess menses bleeding, as it is a specific remedy for causing uterine contractions and stopping the bleeding. An aid in cases of passive pulmonary, gastric, renal, and intestinal bleeding, and bleeding ulcers. Good for diarrhea and excess gas; settles and relaxes stomach. Can sometimes break a fever, especially in cases of cold or flu that exhibit a chilliness of the skin combined with achiness and sweating. Tonsillitis relief. Oral Candida if used as a mouthwash. Lowers the sugar spike that happens after eating, so it is helpful for diabetics.

Parts Used: Bark (cinnamon sticks)

Constituents: Volatile oils, mucilage, diterpenes, proanthocyanidins.

Dosage: Standard infusion using crushed cinnamon sticks, 2 to 4 ounces up to 4 times daily.

Notes: During the Middle Ages, cinnamon was a popular choice for preserving meats. Its antifungal and antibacterial properties helped keep meat from rotting. And if it was rotting already, it masked the awful stench. (Do not try this at home, kids.)

Warnings: Not to be used during pregnancy or breastfeeding. Should not be used in large doses or continual use, as some studies have shown it to become narcotic in doses over 2 grams of cinnamon. To be extra safe, use it when you need it, don't when you don't.

Cleavers (*Galium aparine*)

Uses: A simple diuretic helpful in cases of acute cystitis and/or urethritis with fever and systemic infections. Painful urination combined with infections and fever. Bedwetting in children. Works well as a blood purifier; helps clear swollen lymph glands. Ovarian cysts. Prostate issues such as benign prostatic hypertrophy (BPH). Skin problems such as psoriasis, eczema, hives, scarlet fever, etc. Mononucleosis. Fevers, although it's not a diaphoretic. Nervous, itchy individuals. Underarm odor. Fibrous breasts with numerous cysts. Neurological disease. Dupuytren's contracture. Morton's neuroma.

Parts Used: Whole above-ground plant

Constituents: Coumarins, iridoid glycosides, tannins, citric acid, gallotannic acid.

Dosage: Cold or standard infusion. As needed.

Notes: Cleavers are one of those plants I enjoy hunting for in the woods during the springtime. They have a wonderful flavor that many people like to add to salads, although I'd rather just crunch it freshly picked. Cleavers are also fun for kids. Why? Pick a piece and throw it at someone. It will literally cleave to their shirt! Nature's Velcro.

Warnings: None known.

Corn Silk (*Zea mays*)

Uses: Inflammation and painful irritation of the urinary tract in infants, children, and adults. Especially helpful with urinary tract inflammation due to a bacterial infection. Incontinence and bedwetting. Kidney stones with inflammation and pain. Water retention relief due to kidney and heart issues. Good aid for children with renal issues.

Parts Used: Stigmas

Constituents: Potassium salts, allantoin, sterols, hordenine, tannins, saponins, flavonoids, lipids, glucids, glycoproteins, cryptoxanthin, anthocyanins, plant acids, vitamins C and sometimes K.

Dosage: Standard infusion, 4 to 6 ounces up to 3 times daily.

Notes: Corn Silk is that long hair-like stuff you pull off a fresh ear of corn and throw away. While you can certainly keep and dry the silk for use in tea, it should only be done if you know the corn is organic. I'd recommend purchasing organic even if you buy it already dried and packaged for tea.

Warnings: Occasionally, someone will have an allergy to being around corn silk. If you're taking Lasix (furosemide), don't use corn silk. Otherwise considered very safe for adults and children alike.

Cramp Bark *(Viburnum opulus, trilobum)*

Uses: A uterine sedative and tonic, it eases menstrual pain, uterus inflammation, and menstrual cramping that extends into the intestines and legs. Nausea due to painful menstruation. Mittelschmerz (the cramping experienced between periods that often feels like a jab or a poke around the ovaries). A good choice for a woman who endures terrible cramping every month. Labor, Braxton-Hicks. Threatened miscarriage with cramping; quiets contractions. Good for women who have already experienced a series of miscarriages. Uterine sedative.

Vomiting due to pregnancy. Postpartum pains. Hemorrhage during labor and post-partum. Respiratory spasms due to bronchitis, asthma, and whooping cough. Also good for musculoskeletal spasms.

Parts Used: Root bark, bark

Constituents: Hydroquinones, coumarins, tannins.

Dosage: Cold infusion or strong decoction, 2 to 5 ounces up to 3 times daily.

Notes: For women who have suffered a series of miscarriages, cramp bark is a good tea to use. Whenever that familiar twinge hits, have a tea. Also excellent for very hard and painful periods. If the experience is painful every month, it's important to find out why. But while searching for the cause, cramp bark brings relief.

Warnings: If using during pregnancy, take in moderation. Consult your physician or midwife before consuming.

D

Dandelion *(Taraxacum officinale)*

Uses: An excellent spring tonic and blood thinner. Fresh whole spring-harvested plant provides electrolyte balance and works as a wonderful diuretic that doesn't deplete the system of potassium. Cleanses blood. Good for someone who has a white coated tongue, either solid or patchy. Bronchitis. Indigestion. High blood pressure. High cholesterol. Diabetes type II; hypoglycemia. Kidney infections, achy kidneys that are relieved after urination. PMS. Mastitis or breast congestion. Menopause when combined with poor liver function. Rheumatoid arthritis. Skin issues such as eczema, acne, boils, herpes. Canker sores. Jaundice, hepatitis. Constipation with mouth sores. Shigellosis. Acne with mouth sores. Gout. Fall-harvested root is good as a mild laxative, especially when constipation is combined with a frontal headache, hemorrhoids, or biliousness.

Parts Used: Whole plant; roots, leaves, flowers.

Constituents: Sesquiterpene lactones, diterpenes, inulin, aesculin, eudesmanolides, germacranolides, sterols, triterpenes, carotenoids, flavonoids, polysaccharides. Potassium in the greens.

Dosage: Strong decoction of the root, 2 to 4 ounces up to 4 times daily. Standard infusion of the leaf, 3 to 6 ounces as needed.

Notes: Dandelion root can be roasted and ground, then used as a coffee substitute. It's nice combined with roasted ground chicory root or brewed on its own.

Warnings: None known.

Dill (*Anethum graveolens*)

Uses: Excellent remedy for flatulence due to colic, especially in children. Stimulates lactation. Good for tummy upset. Mild antibacterial action.

Parts Used: Seed

Constituents: Volatile oil, flavonoids, coumarins, xanthone derivatives, triterpenes, phenolic acids, protein, fixed oil.

Dosage: Standard infusion, 2 to 4 ounces up to 4 times daily.

Notes: In the August 2005 edition of the *Journal of Agricultural and Food Chemistry*, it was announced that dill is able to stop the growth of bacteria, yeast, and molds. While they did not confirm it, it's also been suspected of being delicious in pickles.

Warnings: None known.

E

Echinacea *(Echinacea purpurea, angustifolia)*

Uses: Excels as an immunostimulant, blood purifier, lymphatic cleanser. Antiviral, antibacterial, antibiotic. Cold, flu, viruses, infections, fevers, allergies. Strep throat. Tonsillitis. Laryngitis, pharyngitis. Acute sinusitis. Humid asthma with cough. Septic diarrhea. Toxic albuminuria. Eczema, skin ulcers, edema, boils, carbuncles, psoriasis, hives, etc. Septicemia, septic infections. Mouth inflammation in nursing infants. Infant teething (tea rubbed on the gums). Mononucleosis. Also stimulates growth of connective tissue, heals damaged tissues. Venomous bites, stings from insects, snakes.

Parts Used: Root

Constituents: Heterotri-and-heterotetraglycans, echinacein, echinolone, echinoside, echinacin B, sesquiterpenes, diterpenes, inulin, two isomeric 2-methyltetradecadienes, caffeic acid.

Dosage: Standard infusion, ½ to 1 tsp. ground root steeped in 1 cup water, up to 4 times daily.

Notes: Not long ago and against my better judgment, I ended up with an injured baby squirrel. The youngster's nest had been attacked by a hawk, the baby getting a nasty puncture wound on his shoulder. As one can imagine, his health quickly declined. After a few days of caring for him, I realized that the wound was infected, as hawks are not known for having very hygienic talons. In a last ditch effort, I gave the squirrel echinacea tincture, and he turned around remarkably well. For one full day, he went from limp and panting to racing in the grass and hopping around bright-eyed. Unfortunately, I didn't start the echinacea soon enough to save him from the septicemia, but the experience left an indelible impression on me, as to what healing powers this plant contains.

Warnings: There is some concern about AIDS and leukemia patients using the herb, although I've also read plenty of information stating it's safe. If you have an auto-immune disease, it's best to consult your physician before use.

Elder Flower (*Sambucus spp.*)

Uses: Excellent simple herb for fevers, cold, flu, chronic sinusitis, croup. Also for bronchitis, as it clears bronchial phlegm. Edema. Skin issues brought on by metabolic toxins; weeping skin dermatitis, such as from poison ivy and poison oak. A great choice for children. Simple diuretic for the relief of water retention.

Parts Used: Flowers

Constituents: Triterpenes, fixed oils, phenolic acids, pectin, sugars.

Dosage: Standard infusion, 2 to 4 ounces up to 3 times daily.

Notes: This is a beautiful ancient remedy which is safe for children as well as adults, and it seems to do an especially nice job with children. Blend it with equal amounts of peppermint and yarrow for even more cold and flu relief. If you're seen with elder, beware of people quoting Monty Python in your presence: "Your mother was a hamster and your father wreaked of elderberries." Tough words, indeed.

Warnings: If you're fortunate enough to have access to fresh elder, make sure you don't eat the fresh berries, leaves, flowers, etc. While the cooked berries and the dried flowers steeped for tea are wonderfully safe remedies for all ages, the plant in its raw state can cause nausea, vomiting, diarrhea, tachycardia, convulsions, etc.

Elecampane *(Inula helenium)*

Uses: Chronic bronchitis, humid bronchial asthma, acute cough, pneumonia. Good expectorant for any coughing issue with lots of mucous. Tuberculosis, emphysema, silicosis. Whooping cough. Respiratory infections, especially those that cause indigestion due to excess mucous. Chronic mucous discharge from the urinary bladder. Endometriosis, delayed menses, amenorrhea. Appetite stimulant.

Parts Used: Root

Constituents: Inulin, helenin, eudesmanolides, essential oil containing alantolactone (elecampane camphor).

Dosage: Strong decoction, 4 to 6 ounces up to 3 times daily.

Notes: Elecampane is a beautiful plant and makes showy yellow flowers that are a nice addition to a medicinal herb garden. The roots have a strong camphor-like scent due to the alantolactone, or elecampane camphor. The first time I tried this tea I thought it stank, then I liked it, then I wrinkled up my nose, then I smelled it again. Now I like the smell. It means relief!

Warnings: Not to be used during pregnancy. In very large doses, it may cause vomiting and diarrhea.

Eleuthero Root
also called
Siberian Ginseng (*Eleutherococcus senticosus*)

Uses: Early stages of multiple sclerosis or in the beginning of remissions. An aid in injury recovery. Adrenal cortex hypofunctions. In arteriosclerosis, it's lipid lowering. Eases acne caused by excessive cortical hormones. Excellent for increasing mental alertness and increasing the body's ability to tolerate stress; boosts performance and stamina. A good tonic for those going through athletic training. Strengthens digestion. Research has been done which shows it aids in cases of atherosclerosis, diabetes, hypertension, hypotension, cancer, and neurosis. Balances out negative effects of radiation therapy and chemotherapy. Chronic fatigue relief. Immune dysfunction syndrome.

Parts Used: Root

Constituents: Eleutherosides A-E; glycosides, including sterols, lignans, and phenolics; polysaccharides.

Dosage: Cold infusion, 2 to 4 ounces up to 3 times daily.

Notes: Formerly called Siberian ginseng, that name was banned in the U.S. by the Ginseng Labeling Act of 2002.

Warnings: Enhances effects of antibiotics and hexobarbital, so check with your health care professional before taking eleuthero if already using either substance.

F

Fennel (*Foeniculum vulgare*)

Uses: Indigestion with flatulence. Colic with flatulence in infants. Suppressed lactation, particularly when stress induced. Indigestion, fullness after meals, stomach cramps. Nausea. Food poisoning. Coughs and colds. Lung congestion, bronchitis, emphysema, asthma, and shortness of breath.

Parts Used: Seed

Constituents: Volatile oil, anethole, fenchone, flavonoids, coumarins, sterols, fixed oils, sugars.

Dosage: Standard infusion as needed.

Notes: If you're in a pinch and have fennel seed in your spice cupboard, that'll work just fine unless it's really old. (Kitchen spice cupboards are notorious for housing ancient bottles of herbs. I think my mother still has some that came in a spice rack received as a wedding gift in 1966! Don't tell her I told you. Oh, drat. She reads all my stuff.)

Warnings: Consult your physician or midwife before taking during pregnancy.

Feverfew *(Chrysanthemum parthenium)*

Uses: Excellent relief for migraine headaches, as it's anti-inflammatory and antispasmodic. Sometimes helps with arthritis when acute inflammation is present. Relief of menstrual cramps and pain. Stomachaches, toothaches. Lupus. Rheumatoid arthritis.

Parts Used: Whole above-ground herb

Constituents: Sesquiterpene   lactones,   onoterpenes, sesquiterpenes, flavonoids.

Dosage: Cold infusion, 2 to 4 ounces up to 4 times daily.

Notes: Feverfew is another great garden herb. It tolerates a lot and doesn't need any attention, really, which makes it a great choice for my own neglected garden. The fastest way to get the migraine action on this one is to go chew a fresh leaf or two. This will work much faster than any pill you can swallow, and I've experienced the speed myself. The fresh leaf is extremely bitter, but if you enjoy dark chocolate, you can come around to liking the taste of bitter herbs like feverfew.

Warnings: Do not use during pregnancy or while taking anticoagulants or anti-inflammatory medication. Not to be used if blood disorders are present.

G

Ginger (*Zingiber officinalis*)

Uses: Beginning of a head cold with chills and/or a cough. Flu relief. Brings on a sweat and breaks a dry fever. Arteriosclerosis paired with confusion. Diarrhea, dysentery, indigestion, flatulence with painful intestinal spasms. Increases bile secretion and the activity of digestive enzymes. Relieves menstruation with pain. Morning sickness, motion sickness. Improves circulation, thus providing relief for people who are always chilly; chilly hands, feet. Brew it with coffee for effective hangover relief.

Parts Used: Root

Constituents: Volatile oils such as zingiberol, zingiberene, gingerol, shogaol, phellandrene, borneol, cineole; also citral, starch, mucilage, and resin.

Dosage: Strong decoction, 1 to 2 ounces as needed.

Notes: You can usually find fresh ginger root for sale in grocery stores. It works best in its fresh form, so just peel and grate or chop before decoction. If you purchase it organic (always best), you don't have to be too fastidious about peeling it. This is a good remedy for all and is safe for young children and the elderly.

Warnings: Do not use if you have gastric ulcers. Safe for use during pregnancy but in low, responsible doses.

Ginkgo (*Ginkgo biloba*)

Uses: Arteriosclerosis; in the elderly combined with dizziness. It's also a cerebral vasodilator which enhances mental astuteness and aids in concentration and memory. May help in Alzheimer's with depression. Helps relieve dizziness and vertigo, such as that experienced during an attack of Meniere's disease. Also relieves chronic inflammation in the ears and tinnitus and is an aid in cases of cochlear deafness. Asthma. Migraines. Cold hands and feet. Male erectile dysfunction due to poor circulation. Leg ulcers, hemorrhoids, varicose veins. Also good for diabetic retinopathy, retinal insufficiency, macular degeneration, Raynaud's disease, diabetic skin lesions, cataracts, intermittent limping, and varicose veins.

Parts Used: Leaves

Constituents: Terpene lactones, ginkgolide A, B, C, and J; bilobalide and quercetin, kaempferol and isohamnetin.

Dosage: Standard Infusion, 2 to 4 ounces up to 4 times daily.

Notes: After the Chernobyl disaster, ginkgo was used heavily as an aid against radiation-induced injuries.

Warnings: Not to be used in cases of hemophilia. May also prevent ovulation.

Ginseng or American Ginseng (*Panax quinquefolium*)

Uses: In arteriosclerosis, it's lipid lowering. Early stages of multiple sclerosis, or beginning of remissions. Acne caused by excessive cortical hormones. Delay of first menses in young girls who've had a recent growth spurt. Sterility, low sperm count. Anorexia nervosa; especially good for anorexia caused by cancer treatments. Good in cases of nervous exhaustion, as it nourishes and tones the adrenals. Normalizes blood pressure. Decreases blood cholesterol. Helps modify stress levels within the body. Enhances stamina, cognitive function, memory.

Parts Used: Leaves

Constituents: Acetic acid, adenine, adenosine, alanine, ascorbic acid, benzoic acid, beta-sitosterol, caryophyllene, cysteine, ferulic acid, folic acid, at least 10 ginsenosides, glycine, guanidine, histidine, Isoleucine, kaempferol, magnesium, malic acid, niacin, pantothenic acid, salicylic acid, tannins, tyrosine, vanadium, zinc.

Dosage: Cold infusion, 2 to 4 ounces up to 3 times daily.

Notes: American ginseng is endangered, so be sure to purchase it from a reputable source. There are growers in the U.S. who can provide you with responsibly produced root. I've provided info for purchasing in the Herbal Shopping Guide at the end of this book.

Warnings: Not to be used when taking the drug Phenelzine, as manic-like symptoms may result. It also may not be a good choice for people with bipolar disorders. Check with your health care professional first.

Golden Seal (*Hydrastis canadensis*)

Uses: Helpful remedy for colds and flu, sore throats. Acute or chronic middle ear infections. Good for conjunctivitis if used as an eyewash. Stimulates mucous secretions and is antibiotic, therefore is helpful with particularly mucousy head colds, chronic sinusitis, and rhinitis. Relieves bronchial phlegm. Chronic anorexia. Chronic colic. Dysentery recuperation. Acute or chronic gastritis and recuperation. Chronic atonic indigestion and weak digestion. Chronic ulceration and colitis. Vaginitis. Hemorrhoids. Nausea from too much alcohol the night before. Herpes simplex. Leucorrhea. Aids in convalescence after a long period of fever or inflammation.

Parts Used: Leaf

Constituents: Berberine, hydrastine, fatty acids, resin, phenylpropanoids, phytosterins, small amounts of volatile oil.

Dosage: Standard infusion, 1 to 3 ounces up to 4 times daily.

Notes: It's common for the root to be used for medicinal purposes, but it's not very water soluble. As a tea, the leaves are used. Since golden seal is a protected plant which has been heavily harvested in the wild, learning to use the leaves is definitely beneficial both for you and the plant's existence. Always purchase it from a responsible source, such as the ones listed at the end of this book.

Warnings: Pregnant women should consult a qualified health care professional before use.

Ground Ivy (*Glechoma hederacea*)

Uses: Primary use is for the inner ear in cases of tinnitus, hearing loss, buzzing or humming noises, etc. Also useful for the middle ear when irritated by head colds or in chronic respiratory congestion when the Eustachian tubes are blocked. GI problems with griping pains and gas. Relieves mouth sores when used as a gargle. Jaundice caused by stoppage in the gallbladder or liver. Congested spleen and lymphatics. Blood thinner. Sciatica, hip gout, arthritis in hands and knees.

Endocrine conditions such as premature aging. Traditional cancer remedy. Spasms due to fever. Can be used externally for skin eruptions. Used to remove heavy metals and even petrochemical pollutants from the body.

Parts Used: Leaf

Constituents: Rosmarinic acid, methyl isoferuloyl-7-(3,4-dihydroxyphenyl) lactate (1), benzyl-4'-hydroxy-benzoyl-3'O-B-D-glucopyranoside (4).

Dosage: Standard infusion, 1 to 3 ounces up to 4 times daily.

Notes: Ground ivy is a common lawn and garden "weed" which can be harvested when you're certain you can recognize it. Never gather it from the side of a house or structure, and never pick any that has come into contact with lawn fertilizers, pesticides, etc. Always make sure you gather it from a clean source. I like to get mine from my organic vegetable garden. Then I can avoid weeding and just say it's medicine.

Warnings: None known.

H

Hawthorne (*Crataegus spp.*)

Uses: Brings a general overall health to the heart, including muscular tone. A fantastic heart tonic that is good for degenerative heart disease, arteriosclerosis, myocarditis, and a nervous heart with palpitations. Aids with any heart weaknesses due to infectious disease, debilitating disease, smoker's heart, etc. Good for those with high blood pressure. Angina pectoris and arteriosclerosis also find support in hawthorne. Also aids in cases of sudden terror or when there's a deep-seated looming fear of impending doom, etc. Relieves pain in the heart due to strenuous activities one may not be accustomed to doing. Sensation of heart skipping a beat, heart palpitations due to stimulants, arrhythmias in general. Tightness in chest.

Parts Used: Dried berries

Constituents: Flavonoids; vitexin; quercetin; hyperoside; rutin; oligomeric procyanidins; triterpene, ursolic, oleanolic, crataegolic, and phenolic acids.

Dosage: Cold infusion, 1 to 2 ounces up to 2 times daily.

Notes: There are so many variations on the hawthorne that even botanists can't always identify which species is before them. Some are trees, some bushes (the hawthorne, not the botanists), but the good news is they all work interchangeably. (Again, the hawthorne, not the botanists.)

Warnings: Not to be used during pregnancy.

Horehound (*Marrubium vulgare*)

Uses: An effective expectorant helpful for dry coughs and hacking. Also a respiratory sedative that relaxes the bronchioles, making it a good aid for humid asthma, especially when the asthma attack is brought on by allergies. Chronic bronchitis, sinusitis, whooping cough, shortness of breath, colds, flu. Chronic respiratory phlegm. Laryngitis, hoarseness. Brings on suppressed menses. Drink cold and weak to relieve stomachache and colic. Use externally for skin ulcers, dog bites, and shingles.

Parts Used: Flowering herb

Constituents: Diterpene lactones, marrubiin, premarrubiin, diterpene alcohols, volatile oil, flavonoids, alkaloids, choline, alkanes, phytosterols, tannins.

Dosage: Cold infusion, 2 to 4 ounces up to 4 times daily.

Notes: Horehound is a good remedy for children, although I can't promise they'll enjoy the taste. Lots of honey added to the tea will make it more palatable, even blending it with some licorice root, which is naturally sweet and also good for coughing and asthma in children. When I was a girl, my father and grandfather loved horehound candy, and I liked to cajole them into give me some. I think they just thought it was funny I liked it. Maybe I didn't at first and just wanted to be like them, but to this day, the taste of horehound brings back pleasant memories. And these days I truly like it.

Warnings: Not for extended use, as it may cause hypertension in some, particularly the elderly. Can cause irregular heartbeat in some people. In large doses it has a laxative effect. Not to be used during pregnancy.

Horsetail (*Equisetum arvense*)

Uses: This herb has a high silica content, making it good for healing scar tissue associated with emphysema and asthma. Tuberculosis remedy. It also adds elasticity and strength to the alveolar sacs in the lungs and the nephron tubules of the kidneys. Aids in acute cystitis or urethritis. Nighttime incontinence, either that brought on by cystitis or in older males who have an enlarged prostate. Also for incontinence in children accompanied by nightmares. Repairs connective tissue, thus a good aid for osteoporosis and arthritic joint erosion. Rheumatoid arthritis relief. Edema. A diuretic herb. Nourishing to the bones, hair, cartilage, skin, and mucous membranes.

Parts Used: Whole above-ground plant

Constituents: Silica, potassium, manganese, alkaloids, flavonoids, sterols, phenolic acids, organic acids, saponins.

Dosage: Standard decoction followed by 15 minutes of steeping before removal of herb. Drink 1 to 2 times daily.

Notes: Due to its high silica and mineral content, horsetail is indeed strengthening to the hair, nails, and teeth. But always make sure you have Equisetum arvense and not any other form of horsetail.

Warnings: I highly advise you get organic horsetail. If the herb is gathered downstream from factories or agricultural areas, it can contain heavy levels of toxins. Do not ingest the herb itself. Make the tea and throw away the strained herb, as it can irritate the GI tract.

Hyssop *(Hyssopus officinalis)*

Uses: Skin abrasions and bruises when applied topically. Also good for muscle pain when applied topically. Antiviral and antispasmodic which is helpful with bronchitis, asthma, and croupy coughs. A diaphoretic, it brings on sweating in a dry fever. An old-time remedy for cold, flu, and bronchial infection; good for any age. A trustworthy, relaxing anti-inflammatory for children. Tonsillitis, sore throat, swollen glands. Hoarseness. Nervine properties make it an anxiety remedy. Bright's disease, kidney infection, edema. Can be used externally for fibromyalgia. Infantile paralysis.

Parts Used: Flowering herb

Constituents: Diterpenes, triterpenoid saponins, volatile oil, flavonoids, hysopin, tannins, resin.

Dosage: Standard infusion, 6 to 8 ounces up to 3 times daily.

Notes: Hyssop used to be viewed as a cure-all and was highly esteemed in the world of medicinal herbs. Today, it is often overlooked and shouldn't be. It's also a great garden herb that's weather resistant and attractive to bees and butterflies.

Warnings: Not to be used during pregnancy.

J

Juniper (*Juniperus communis*)

Uses: Chronic non-inflamed cystitis or urethritis. Non-inflamed prostatitis. Painful urination after a hysterectomy. Diuretic and stimulant for the stomach. Chronic arthritis, gout, muscular rheumatic disease. Flatulence. Poor digestion, appetite in atonic digestive systems. Relieves pain and inflammation in arthritis and gout.

Parts Used: Berries (most effective) or leaves

Constituents: Volatile oil, myrcene, sabinene, a- and b-pinene, 4-cineole, camphene, limonene, condensed tannins, diterpenes, flavonoids, sugars, resin, vitamin C.

Dosage: Standard infusion of berries, 2 to 3 ounces up to 3 times daily. Standard infusion of leaves, 2 to 4 ounces up to 3 times daily.

Notes: Juniper berries have a very long history of medicinal use dating to the ancient Egyptians. Back in 1500 B.C., it was the tapeworm remedy of choice. Lots of cultures thought it was good for warding off evil. If you consider flatulence evil, then I guess they were right.

Warnings: Short-term use only. May irritate the kidneys over time. If you've been using it awhile and your urine starts smelling like violets, this means you've used the tea too long. It does not mean you have magical urine.

K

Kava Kava (*Piper methysticum*)

Uses: Relaxing to the central nervous system, it brings a peace and calm to an anxiety-filled person. Also good in cases of despondency, nervousness, or depression. Supportive to those with tremors due to Parkinson's disease and the like. Pain in the top or the back of the eyeball. Neuralgia in the middle ear. Pain relief for cystitis, urethritis, and pain in urination. Ulcers that awaken at night with pain. Prostatitis paired with urethritis. Insomnia. Fibromyalgia. Attention deficit hyperactivity disorder (ADHD). PMS relief, painful menstruation. It can be used topically as an antifungal for athlete's foot, ringworm, etc.

Parts Used: Root

Constituents: Kavalactones, methysticin, dihydromethysticin, kavain, dihydrokavain, chalcones.

Dosage: Standard infusion, 4 to 8 ounces up to 2 times daily.

Notes: There is a lot of misunderstanding surrounding kava. There was quite a bit of hoopla in the media several years back stating it was dangerous, but responsible herbalists the world over don't agree. Yes, it's true you don't want to sit down to several cups. You'll probably barf. But then you'll be fine. And yes, it's true drinking alcohol and then having a cup of kava tea will also make you barf. But then you'll be fine, right after swearing to never go out drinking again. My best advice is to remember that just because one cup of kava tea feels really nice, that doesn't mean two or three is going to feel great. It won't. Trust me.

Warnings: Not to be used during pregnancy or while nursing. Should not be used with alcohol. Do not use in large amounts, as it may impair your ability to drive and operate heavy machinery.

L

Lavender (*Lavandula officinalis*)

Uses: Colic or indigestion, including nervous indigestion, with flatulence. Nausea. Motion sickness. Severe headaches, migraines. Tension in neck and shoulder area. Colic in infants, paired with nausea and sour breath. Acidic vomiting in children. Flu relief, bronchitis, asthma, whooping cough. Nervousness, anxiousness, dizziness, fainting spells, depression, worry, sleeplessness, nightmares. While it relaxes, it also enhances mental acuteness.

Parts Used: Flowers

Constituents: Volatile oil, coumarins, triterpenes, flavonoids.

Dosage: Standard infusion, 2 to 3 ounces up to 4 times daily.

Notes: This is a lovely remedy for colic in infants and can even be used before the mother's milk has come in, if needed.

If the infant won't take the tea in a bottle, either apply the tea to the mother's nipples before feeding, or dribble some tea into the infant's mouth by first dipping a bit of clean cotton into the tea. See Clark's Rule at the end of this book for the proper dosage for your infant or child.

Warnings: None known.

Lemon Balm (*Melissa officinalis*)

Uses: Relaxes the neurons and lowers stress while elevating the mood when depressed. Smoothes you out while not making you feel druggy. Cools the body down on hot days. Mild sedative, antispasmodic. Antiviral effect that is good for herpes; shortens the outbreak and reduces the pain. Also anti-inflammatory and antioxidant. Relieves chills and fevers. Blues due to PMS. Great for infants and young children, especially in cases of cold, flu, fevers, teething, nervousness, sleeplessness, peevishness. Stomach pain, diarrhea, gastroenteritis, intestinal gas, and severe menstrual cramps all find relief in this herb.

Parts Used: Flowering herb

Constituents: Flavonoids, rosmarinic acid, ferulic acid, caffeic acid, methyl carnosoate, hydroxycinnamic acid, and 2-(3',4'-dihydroxyphenyl)-1,3-benzodioxole-5-aldehyde.

Dosage: Standard infusion as needed.

Notes: This is an easy herb to grow yourself. If you harvest your own, the prime time to do it is on a mid to late spring morning before the sun is full power. Water the plant the night before, and only pick in the morning after the dew is gone. Try not to touch the leaves while bundling. Dry them in a brown paper bag. Lemon balm doesn't stay fresh for long, so harvest the leaves every spring and toss out the old stuff.

Warnings: None known.

Licorice (*Glycyrrhiza glabra*)

Uses: Acute coughs, chronic bronchitis, laryngitis, pharyngitis. Hypotension with frequent urination. Urinary tract irritations. Chronic constipation. Dry bowel movements. Irritable bowel syndrome (IBS) where constipation is the more

105

dominant symptom. Soothes peptic and duodenal ulcers. Strengthening in cases of adrenal exhaustion. States of immune deficiency. Liver inflammation, hepatitis. Licorice sticks (dried root which looks like a twig) can be chewed for teething relief. Some people even find that chewing the licorice sticks helps take the edge off quitting smoking.

Parts Used: Root

Constituents: Glycyrrhizin, hispaglabrin-A and -B, glabridin, isoprenylchalone, licochalcone A, isoliquiritigenin, formononetin, licopyranocoumarin, licoarylcoumarin, glisoflavone, glicoricone, licofuranone.

Dosage: Strong decoction, 1 to 3 ounces up to 3 times daily.

Notes: Licorice is the most popular medicinal herb used in Traditional Chinese Medicine (TCM) and is currently included in over 5,000 Chinese herbal formulas. In fact, it's popular worldwide and is a top medicinal herb in Western herbalism as well. And it makes a darned good jelly bean.

Warnings: May cause sodium retention. Should not be used for more than six weeks at a time without being under the supervision of a health care professional. Not good for those with high blood pressure, heart failure, left ventricular hypertrophy, cirrhosis of the liver, cholestatic liver disorders, and kidney disease. If you use an asthma inhaler or steroids, licorice will increase the medicines' effectiveness and side effects.

M

Marshmallow (*Althea officinalis*)

Uses: Astringent to the mucosa and tissues. Head cold with laryngitis or hoarse throat, viral infections, urinary tract infections, and urinary tract stress. Dry mouth, throat, laryngitis, pharyngitis (use as gargle). Bronchitis, asthma, whooping cough, emphysema. Cystitis, urethritis. Stomach ulcer relief. Diarrhea relief. Sometimes used during chemotherapy as a support. Immune stimulant with properties that appear to be close to echinacea. Anti-inflammatory.

Parts Used: Root

Constituents: Polysaccharides, mucilage, asparagine, tannins.

Dosage: Cold infusion as needed.

Notes: If you've gone through a course of antibiotics but you're still not feeling completely well, make up some marshmallow tea (cold infusion, 1 ounce herb to 1 quart water) and keep it refrigerated. Continue to drink 3 or 4 cups of it for a week, just to get you through the last of what you've been dealing with.

Before purchasing your marshmallow root, smell it first if you're able. The old root will have a sort of vinegar smell to it and should be avoided. Drinking it won't be very pleasant, either. I can tell you from personal experience that there's a big difference in taste. I won't touch old marshmallow with a 10-foot pole.

Warnings: None known.

Motherwort (*Leonurus cardiaca*)

Uses: Brings on suppressed menstruation, especially when tension or anxiety are being experienced. May ease false labor pains. Good to ease tension during menopause. Relieves the stress, cramping, and pain of PMS; also reduces headaches and cravings related to PMS. A wonderful heart tonic that strengthens the heart without straining it. Anxiety, tension, fear, panic attacks with heart palpitations. Heart skipping a beat when stressed. Hypertension tachycardia. Herpes relief. Good for elevated thyroid.

Parts Used: Flowering herb

Constituents: Iridoids, labdane diterpenes, flavonoids, caffeic acid, alkaloids, tachydrine, betonicine, turicin, leonurine, tannins, volatile oil.

Dosage: Standard infusion, 2 to 4 ounces up to 4 times daily.

Notes: When my son was about four, we were talking about herbs together. He told me that he knew why motherwort had its name. He explained that you take it when you're scared or worried and want your mommy but she's not there. Leave it to a kid to explain things just right!

Warnings: Not to be used during pregnancy. If you are taking prescription medication for your heart, consult your physician or pharmacist before using.

Mullein (*Verbascum thapsus*)

Uses: Excellent as a tonic for asthma and weak lungs; relaxant to the lungs, it works as a bronchial dilator, expanding airways. Brings relief to uncontrollable coughing fits caused by bronchitis, whooping cough, hay fever, allergies, and asthma. Good for hot and tight bronchial infections. Clears lungs after inhalation of smoke, pollution, or toxic dust. Also brings relief to inflamed urinary passages. Cystitis with burning urine. Diarrhea and constipation. Painful and/or bleeding hemorrhoids. Mumps. Facial neuralgia.

Parts Used: Leaves

Constituents: Flavonoids, mucilage, saponins, tannins, volatile oil.

Dosage: Standard infusion, 2 to 4 ounces up to 4 times daily.

Notes: I've taken mullein leaf often for lung congestion. I find that when there's a tightness in the lungs or a buildup of old mucous that just isn't moving, this is a great remedy. Drink some tea, wait awhile, then have some more if the mucous isn't moving yet. Just be forewarned that large amounts of the herb can give you a serious coughing fit that, while it will clear those lungs out, will totally exhaust you afterwards.

Mullein root is one of my favorite herbal teas, although you can't buy the root in commerce. It's probably because it's so darned time consuming to collect and clean. Tea from the root provides a wonderful muscle relaxing effect that helps if something in your spine just feels out of place. Think liquid chiropractor. It's also nice for people who experience the sensation that their brain is "tight." To prepare the root, make 2 to 3 ounces of strong decoction, taken up to 4 times daily.

Warnings: None known.

O

Oak (*Quercus robur, gambelii, alba,* or *fendleri*)

Uses: Strengthens teeth, aids with cavities, tightens loose teeth, freshens bad breath, relieves canker sores, restores bleeding or inflamed gums. Good for bleeding ulcers or internal bruising. Sinus congestion, mucous in the stomach, postnasal drip, and indigestion. Strep throat, tonsillitis. Swollen glands of the throat. Early stages of tuberculosis, builds resistance to tuberculosis. Swollen spleen. Hemorrhoids, intestinal prolapse, diarrhea, dysentery. Bloody urine, cystitis. Vaginitis. Osteoporosis. Use externally for skin ulcers, scratches, abrasions, or acute early stages of herpes. Leaf tea is a blood tonic. Can also be used like quinine to treat a recurring fever with achy limbs and chills. For leaf tea, steep in cold water overnight and use freely.

Parts Used: Any part of the tree may be used: leaves, bark, roots, branches.

Constituents: Tannins, phlobatannin, ellagitannins, gallic acid.

Dosage: Cold infusion for internal use, as needed. Strong decoction for external use.

Notes: The bark is the most commonly used portion of the oak, although herbalists have relied on all parts of the tree throughout history, and many still do. But if you purchase it in commerce, you'll most likely be getting the inner bark. When gathering it on your own, it's easiest to gather the leaves or the inner bark of twigs, and it's safer for the tree.

Warnings: None known.

Oats (*Avena sativa*)

Uses: Relieves chest pains, in particular those brought on by fear. Good for nervous exhaustion, emotional exhaustion. Prevents anxiety surrounding insomnia. General insomnia remedy. Narcolepsy. Jet lag. Menopausal aid for sense of confusion or melancholy. Remedy for PMS jumpiness. Builds up weak appetite. Hysteria. Good nutritive tea. Aids in withdrawal from drugs, smoking, alcohol.

Parts Used: Straw (dry but green)

Constituents: Carbohydrates, silicic acid.

Dosage: Standard infusion, 4 to 8 ounces up to 4 times daily.

Notes: In case you were wondering, rolled oats are not used in the same way, but you can put them in your bath to soothe skin irritation like hives and eczema. Or just save them for cookies and homemade granola. That's nice, too.

Warnings: None known.

Ox-Eye Daisy *(Chrysanthemum leucanthemum)*

Uses: Rebuilds after a fever, in particular a fever with excessive sweating. Excellent for relieving a runny nose, especially when brought on by allergies, hay fever, or the beginning of a head cold. An anti-inflammatory. Whooping cough, asthma, chronic coughs. Nervousness. Night sweats.

Parts Used: Flowering herb

Constituents: Essential oils, tannins, saponins, mucilage, flavones.

Dosage: Standard infusion, 4 to 8 ounces up to 4 times daily.

Notes: This is an overlooked but highly useful herb. Ox-eye daisies grow in proliferation all over much of the U.S. and Europe. They're effective for opening up the sinuses, yet they're hardly ever mentioned in herbal guides or sold in commerce. I added it to the list of 101 only because they're easy to identify (check out wild plant guides and www.eol.org for photos), they're plentiful, and they're often considered an invasive species, which means no one will arrest you for picking them. Unless you're yanking them out of your neighbor's garden or pulling them out of state parks. You can grow it in your own garden too, with much success and little effort.

Warnings: If you are allergic to ragweed, chrysanthemum, marigold, and other related plants, you may be allergic to ox-eye.

Oregon Grape (*Mahonia aquifolium*)

Uses: Does an excellent job in stimulating the protein metabolism of the liver, skin, and mucosa. Helpful herb for those who don't get enough protein in the diet, especially in the elderly. Good choice for liver issues that are paired with dry, cracked skin and brittle hair. Hepatitis, cirrhosis, and jaundice. Eczema, psoriasis, dandruff, acne. Low thyroid with dry skin. Diabetes, sugar cravings. Speeds up the reparation of damaged tissues after injuries, accidents, and disease. Diarrhea, constipation. Dyspepsia from fats; paired with frontal headache and nausea. Nausea after eating, especially after fatty foods. Nausea in general. Chronic indigestion. Motion sickness. Poor appetite. Chronic gastritis from alcoholic excess. Intestinal collapse. Gut infections, colon infections. Congestion of the lymph, swollen glands. PMS that comes with oily skin and a heaviness in the abdomen, and nasty food cravings. Vaginitis. Weak uterus. Allergies, chronic or subacute rhinitis. A good mouthwash for bleeding gums. Hangovers. Great for people who go to the hospital and catch a bug or virus there. It also boosts any antibiotics taken.

Parts Used: Root

119

Constituents: Alkaloids such as berberine, berbamine, hydrastine, oxycanthine.

Dosage: Cold infusion, 1 to 3 ounces up to 3 times daily.

Notes: Oregon grape may sound like the beginnings of a good organic wine, but it's really a kind of barberry. Many herbalists like using it instead of golden seal. It is also used in natural veterinary medicine.

Warnings: None known.

P

Parsley (*Carum petroselinum*)

Uses: Flatulent colic in everyone from infants to adults. A strong diuretic; the seeds are the stronger diuretic of the two, although both root and seed work well. Gravel, stone, congestion of the kidneys. Stimulates the appetite. Freshens bad breath. Improves digestion. Arthritis, gout. Low blood pressure.

Parts Used: Root or seed

Constituents: Volatile oil, coumarins, flavonoids, phthalides, vitamins.

Dosage: Standard infusion of 1 tsp. seeds or 1 Tbs. root to 1 cup water. 1 to 4 times daily.

Notes: Ancient myth claims parsley first came from the spilled blood of Archemorus when he got eaten by serpents. That's just gross.

Warnings: Not to be used during pregnancy due to uterine stimulant effects.

Passionflower (*Passiflora incarnata*)

Uses: A wonderful sedative herb that lowers blood pressure and relieves insomnia. Helpful in cases of evening heart palpitations. Antispasmodic that's useful for those with Parkinson's disease, seizures, and hysteria. Nervous excitement. Also good for long-term use as an antispasmodic for asthma. Relieves nerve pain such as neuralgia and shingles. Anti-inflammatory. Good for insomnia without a "hangover" in the morning.

Parts Used: Whole above-ground plant

Constituents: Alkaloids, flavonoids.

Dosage: Standard infusion, 2 to 6 ounces up to 4 times daily.

Notes: If you've never seen a real passionflower before, be sure to look it up. A gorgeous combination between something from the forests of Avatar and Dr. Seuss's wildest imaginings, there's no wonder it's captivated Central and Southern American herbalists for hundreds of years. I think just looking at it is enough to lull one into a peaceful state.

Warnings: Not to be used with sedative medications. May cause vomiting and overexcitement in children under the age of four.

Pau D'Arco (*Tabebuia impetiginosa*)

Uses: Asthma, in particular that which is humid and paired with chronic Candida. Good for Candida sufferers after taking a round of antibiotic or anti-inflammatory medications. Fights Candida and systemic infections by preventing the Candida enzymes from reproducing. Can be used both internally and externally for fungal infections in general. Chronic gastritis with odorous belching. Eczema caused by Candida. Rheumatoid arthritis. A general remedy for allergies. Antioxidant. Increases red blood cell count. Lymphatic congestion.

Parts Used: Bark

Constituents: Lapachol, lapachone, isolapachone, tannins.

Dosage: Cold infusion, 2 to 4 ounces up to 3 times daily.

Notes: With a long history of medicinal use by the indigenous peoples of South and Central America, our scientific knowledge of pau d'arco is only just beginning. But so far, many of the indigenous uses are panning out to be scientifically accurate, a story we see again and again in the world of herbalism.

Warnings: None known.

Peach (*Amygdalus persica*)

Uses: Chronic gastritis with tender abdomen. Morning sickness. General irritation of the stomach. Diarrhea, dysentery, indigestion, gastritis, nausea. Vomiting in children, paired with green diarrhea. Nervousness, insomnia. Good for children who are prone to overexcitability. When used externally, it relieves hives, allergic reactions, and other skin irritations.

Parts Used: Fresh twigs

Constituents: Cyanogenic glycosides.

Dosage: Cold infusion, 1 to 2 ounces as needed.

Notes: While I'm discussing the use of the twigs here, many herbalists also rely on the leaves, bark, flowers, and the unopened pits. But due to their high levels of cyanide, the opened almond-shaped kernels should not be used.

Warnings: Peach leaves, twigs, and kernel all contain cyanogens. In the average dose of tea, this is fine. But you should not consume large amounts of this herb.

Peppermint (*Mentha piperita*)

Uses: Nausea caused by eating, travel, or pregnancy. For infants, children, or adults, it's good in cases of diarrhea, ulcerative colitis, fever, vomiting, colic, flatulence, indigestion, suppressed sweating in colds and flu. Headache, migraine relief, mental fatigue. Lessens excess mucous. A good tonic for nervousness, anxiety, tension, and hysteria. Relieves hiccoughs. Warms the body. Circulatory stimulant. Relieves muscle tension and spasms. Brings measles eruptions to the surface, therefore aiding in faster recovery.

Parts Used: Whole above-ground plant

Constituents: Phenolic acids; essential oil, most components being menthol, menthone, and menthyl acetate; flavonoids; tannins.

Dosage: Cold or standard infusion as needed.

Notes: One of the more popular herb choices for teas, food, and medicine, peppermint is something every home herbalist should have available. It's also easy to grow in the garden or a pot, so you can be sure you've got plenty of freshly dried herb in store. While I've had good luck keeping dried peppermint fresh and aromatic for two or three years, I think it's best to have a new batch of freshly dried herb each year.

Warnings: During pregnancy, only use peppermint under the guidance of your health care professional. In cases of hiatal hernias or acute gallstones, it is not recommended.

Pine (*Pinus spp.*)

Uses: Good for persistent colds and flu. Good for chronic bronchitis, old sinus infections, lung infections, strep throat, tonsillitis, laryngitis, asthma, whooping cough, croup, and cough in general. Relieves indigestion. Use externally for hemorrhoid relief. Edema relief, as it is diuretic. Chronic neuralgia, rheumatism.

Parts Used: Bark, small twigs

Constituents: Dihydropinosylvin, manoyoxide, pinomyricetin, pinoquercetin, pinoresinol, pinosylvin, strobal, strobol.

127

Dosage: Standard infusion, 2 to 4 ounces up to 3 times daily.

Notes: I always have dried pine twigs on my herb shelf. It's the first thing I grab when coughing or lung viruses set in, and I've found it's especially relieving for the sort of asthma that comes with a tight chest and mucous that won't move. It's more gentle at moving the mucous than some herbs, as it has more of a tendency to liquefy the gunk and get it out without putting you through an exhausting coughing fit.

Warnings: In cases of kidney inflammation, do not take strong pine tea, as the tea will stimulate the kidneys. Frequent use of pine also irritates the kidneys.

Pleurisy Root (*Asclepias tuberosa*)

Uses: Good in cases of acute bronchitis, flu, pneumonia, dry non-spasmodic asthma, acute dry coughs, and other respiratory maladies and infections. Fever reducer, which is also good for feverish infants with dry bronchitis and damp skin. Also eases cold symptoms. Persistent eczema. Chronic rheumatic pain paired with a dry cough, intercostal neuralgia, and chronic indigestion.

Constituents: Cardenolides, flavonoids, friedalin, a- and B-amyrin, lupeol, viburnitol, choline sugars.

Dosage: Cold infusion, 2 to 4 ounces up to 3 times daily.

Notes: Pleurisy root is a milkweed also known as butterfly weed. It's the one that the Monarch butterfly relies on for survival, so if you get Monarchs in your area, it's a wonderful addition to the garden. Hummingbirds and many other species of butterflies appreciate it, too. And the flowers are a stunning fiery orange you'll look forward to seeing each year.

Warnings: Not for use during pregnancy. While you should check with your physician before taking any herb while on prescription medications, it's especially important to do before taking pleurisy root. It may interact with several different medications. If you have liver conditions, don't take it.

Prickly Pear *(Opuntia vulgaris, phaeacantha, compressa, polycantha)*

Uses: Internal bruises. Strengthens capillaries in issues such as chronic colitis, pulmonary problems as in asthma and mild bronchiectasis, chronic vaginitis, diverticulosis, benign prostatic hypertrophy.

Parts Used: Dried flowers

Constituents: Isorhamnetin-3-beta-d-glucoside, isorhamnetin-3,7-diglucoside.

Dosage: Standard infusion, 2 or 3 flowers, strained very well. 2 to 4 ounces up to 2 times daily.

Notes: I was surprised several years ago to see a very large stand of prickly pear alive and well in the Northern U.S., but according to herbalist Michael Moore, it grows as far north as British Columbia. At one point, I tried growing some in my own yard after rescuing a few fallen plants but decided against it after it started ravaging an area my son kept wandering into.

130

I like cacti, but not enough to pull the spines out of my son on a regular basis.

Warnings: None known.

132

R

Ragweed (*Ambrosia artemisiifolia, trifida*)

Uses: Middle ear infection brought on by allergies or rhinitis. Acute allergic rhinitis. Septic diarrhea. Good for children and adults suffering from hay fever with subsequent nose and eye pain, and watery nose and eyes.

Parts Used: Herb

Constituents: Ambrosic acid, artemidifolin, artemisiifolin, coronopilin, cumanin, dihydrocumanin, peruvin, psilostachyin, quercetin-3-glucoside.

Dosage: Standard infusion, 1 to 2 ounces up to 4 times daily.

Notes: It may seem counterintuitive to use ragweed in cases of hay fever or allergies, but it's the pollen that causes these reactions, and not the herb itself. This one is hard to find in commerce, so if you're allergic, have someone else pick it for you (after careful identification, of course).

Warnings: Live plant may induce allergic reactions in some.

Raspberry (*Rubus idaeus*)

Uses: An excellent uterine tonic. Aids with heavy menses that includes a dull, achy abdomen. Helps prevent spotting during pregnancy and assists contractions during labor, lessening a tendency to hemorrhage. Good as a general tonic in the last trimester of pregnancy. Painful menses, especially toward the end when red blood is present. Mildly laxative. Aids in diarrhea and hemorrhoids.

Parts Used: Leaves

Constituents: Flavonoids, tannins, fruit sugar, volatile oil, pectin, citric acid, malic acid.

Dosage: Standard infusion as needed.

Notes: I've seen warnings concerning red raspberry tea usage during pregnancy, but overall it is quite safe. The actual stories surrounding the concerns have more to do with drinking very large quantities with the thought that more must be better. The key, as with all things, is moderation. Drinking gallons of the stuff isn't going to produce a super-duper uterus. A few cups of tea throughout the day is more than sufficient. It's also good to sip at during labor.

Dried raspberry leaf should smell like raspberries. The resulting tea should taste like raspberries. If it doesn't, it's probably old and it won't do much. If it does smell like raspberries, boy, is it delicious! Skip that manufactured raspberry iced chemical tea and make your own. Much better!

Warnings: To be taken in moderation during pregnancy and not to be overdone; best when used during last trimester.

Red Clover (*Trifolium pratense*)

Uses: Good for an acute dry or spasmodic cough; croup, whooping cough, asthma. Malnutrition due to a long illness; used in recuperation, as it is high in minerals. Nice maintenance herb, offering nutrition. Parathyroid imbalances. Nutritional malabsorption. Helpful during cancer as a supportive anti-metastatic. Mild sedative for children. Eases dry tear ducts. Significantly reduces hot flashes in menopausal women.

Parts Used: Flowering herb

Constituents: Isoflavones, other flavonoids, clovamides, coumarins, a galactomannan, resins, minerals, vitamins, phytoalexins.

Dosage: Standard infusion or strong decoction, 4 to 6 ounces up to 3 times daily.

Notes: In Traditional Chinese Medicine (TCM), red clover is used for purifying the blood, to remove toxins, and as a tonic for colds.

Warnings: Not for use during pregnancy or for anyone on blood thinning medication.

Rosemary (*Rosmarinus officinalis*)

Uses: A rubefacient, which means it brings blood to the surface; aids in circulation to the head, strengthens capillaries of the brain. Antioxidant. Soothes the nervous system. Brings depression relief to those suffering from nervous disorders. For suppressed menses brought on by exposure to cold weather. Gas and indigestion relief. Fever, cold, and flu aid; will relieve head and chest pain due to cold and flu. Coughing, lung congestion. Can be used externally for skin rashes and ringworm.

Parts Used: Leaves

Constituents: Volatile oil, flavonoids, rosmarinic acid and other phenolic acids, diterpenes, rosmaricine, triterpenes.

Dosage: Standard infusion, 2 to 4 ounces as needed.

Notes: Rosemary tea is great for many things, but let's not forget it's simply a nice tea for tea's sake. It's one of those herbs that manages to relax and invigorate simultaneously. So if you need a kick in the pants about midday, try rosemary tea

137

instead of a jittery cup o' joe. You'll get the boost you need without the crash you don't.

Warnings: None known.

S

Sage *(Salvia spp.)*

Uses: Contains antimicrobial effects. Laryngitis, tonsillitis. Postnasal drip, colds, runny nose. Helps wean infants from breastfeeding when mother drinks the cool tea and washes breasts with the tea. Slows and stops the milk. When the tea is drunk hot, it stimulates sweating in cases of systemic infections that give the person cold hands and feet with chills. Brings on delayed menses. Hot flashes, night sweats. Use as a gargle for sore throats, and for congested sinuses and Eustachian tubes. Can also be used as a strong, effective analgesic wash for cuts, scratches, and inflamed skin. Chronic diarrhea, dysentery.

Parts Used: Flowering herb

Constituents: Isopimaric acid and related diterpenes, histamine, aromatics.

Dosage: Cold or standard infusion, 2 to 4 ounces up to 3 times daily.

Notes: Sage is a complex herb with so many uses there's no room for them all here. Herbalists agree that it's a valuable medicinal plant. One thing that fascinates me: drink it hot and it stimulates secretions such as saliva, sweating, and mucous production throughout the body. Drink the tea cold and it suppresses those very same secretions. Keep that in mind if you choose to use it.

Warnings: None known.

Sagebrush (*Artemisia tridentata*)

Uses: A powerfully antifungal, antimicrobial herb. Stimulates sweating; breaks fevers when drunk hot and taken in small sips. When taken cold, it stimulates digestion. Can be used as an external wash and is commonly used on animals.

Parts Used: Herb

Dosage: Strong infusion, 1 to 2 ounces sipped slowly.

Notes: Another name for sagebrush is "Mormon tea". Interestingly, it was also once referred to as "whorehouse tea" because it was a common remedy for gonorrhea. This stuff tastes bad but it works. To relieve flu symptoms, you can steep some of the dried herb in some brandy or tequila and sip at it. At least the buzz from the alcohol will compensate for the lousy taste.

Warnings: Not for use during pregnancy. Also not to be used in cases of emphysema or bronchiectasis.

St. John's-wort *(Hypericum perforatum)*

Uses: Has a well-earned reputation of relieving depression and "the blues," as it works as a natural MAO inhibitor. Especially helpful when you find yourself unable to get over grief or a bad experience and you need a pull up out of the dark hole. Also good for seasonal depression, such as is caused by a long, dark winter. Aids in depression that is paired with anger. Relieves neuralgia with muscle twitching. Pain reliever. Also increases capillary strength, bringing aid to hemorrhoids and varicose veins. Antiviral and antibacterial,

141

making it a nice choice for those suffering from ear infections. Also helpful in cases of HIV because it seems to lessen the agitation that is experienced. An anti-inflammatory that is sometimes used in cases of concussions or spinal injuries. Works well as a topical for shingles.

Parts Used: Flowering tops, recently dried

Constituents: Volatile oil, hypericin, hyperforin, bioflavones.

Dosage: Standard infusion, 3 to 6 ounces up to 3 times daily.

Notes: While St. John's-wort does work as a tea, it's not nearly as effective as the tinctured form. If you choose to use it as tea, make sure it's recently dried. Anything older than a year will work but loses its potency.

St. John's-wort isn't for clinical depression. It's more for the up-and-down stuff, for people who get depressed and ticked off simultaneously, and for temporary setbacks that you just need to get yourself out of. Sometimes people take the herb and see results immediately. For others, it takes a while.

Warnings: Over time, St. John's-wort can cause photosensitivity in some people, so beware of spending long days in the sun unprotected.

Saw Palmetto (*Serenoa serrulata*)

Uses: Impotency and frigidity relief, paired with difficult urination. Subacute or chronic enlarged prostate, with or without inflammation; in older men, enlarged prostate with dull ache. Works as a prostate anti-inflammatory. Is often used as a support in cases of prostate cancer. Enlarged uterus. Slow physical and sexual maturation in adolescents. Underdeveloped testes, prostate, breasts, uterus, ovaries. Male baldness. In women, it's helpful in cases where there is excessive body hair and/or underdeveloped breasts. May be helpful with polycystic ovaries and ovarian cysts. Relieves chronic bladder infections.

Parts Used: Berries

Constituents: Oleic acid, lauric acid, myristic acid, palmitic acid, beta-sitosterol, campesterol, stigmasterol, cycloartenol, free fatty alcohols, monoglycerides, polysaccharides, essential oil, fixed oil.

Dosage: Standard infusion, 2 to 4 ounces up to 3 times daily.

Notes: For prostate health, it's best to view saw palmetto as an aid that you use in conjunction with other healthy measures. Being sedentary, bicycling a lot, etc., can also degenerate prostate health. So changes of lifestyle may need to be made. Saw palmetto shouldn't be relied on as the prostate cure-all.

Warnings: In very few individuals, it may cause nausea or stomach complaints when taken in large doses.

Senna (*Cassia spp.*)

Uses: A reliable laxative. Relieves chronic constipation and hard feces. It's a good herb to relieve constipation when you suffer from hemorrhoids and need to go easy on the tissues.

Parts Used: Leaves

Constituents: Anthraquinone glycosides, naphthalene glycosides, mucilage, flavonoids, volatile oil, sugars, resins.

Dosage: Standard infusion. Combine ¾ tsp. senna to ¼ tsp. coriander (as an antispasmodic). 4 to 8 ounces before bedtime for morning results.

Notes: Senna is pretty much a one-trick pony. Its thing is getting you out of a "bind" and helping to move the stool. It works by stimulating peristalsis, so if you rely on it too often to go potty, you may find you've paralyzed your peristalsis muscles. That's not a permanent situation and can be reversed by discontinuing the herb, but it's not fun to get off of once you've gotten hooked. Not a daily use herb.

Warnings: Not to be used during pregnancy or if breast feeding. Can be addictive, so only use when you need it. Do not rely on it for regularity.

Shepherd's Purse (*Capsella bursa-pastoris*)

Uses: Remedy to stop a bloody nose. Chronic cystitis or urethritis with scanty or dark urine. Bleeding hemorrhoids, ulcers. Good for blood in urine if the bleeding is not due to serious causes such as cancer. Astringent to the urinary tract. A diuretic for arthritis. Strengthens the effects of oxytocin. Post-partum hemorrhage, menstrual hemorrhage. Placental delivery aid after birthing. Impending miscarriage showing moderate spotting. Good for cases of Braxton Hicks. A good hemostatic for after C-sections, DNC's, and other surgeries. Good for heavy periods that produce a lot of bright red blood and don't seem to slow down, or in cases of fibroids or mid-cycle bleeding.

Parts Used: Whole plant, recently dried

Constituents: Luteolin 7-rutinoside, quercetin 3-rutinoside, bursinic acid, fumaric acid, tyramine, choline.

Dosage: Standard infusion, 2 to 4 ounces up to 4 times daily.

Notes: For hemorrhoids that bleed due to scraping, you can use the tea as an enema. It works very well if you can retain the enema for a few moments before expelling it. (Slow, long-term oozing can be cared for in the same way with cinnamon tea.)

Warnings: May stimulate contractions in pregnancy but can be used in small quantities and under the supervision of a health care professional familiar with the plant. Shouldn't be used at all in cases of bleeding during pregnancy in the seventh month or later, as it can slightly stimulate oxytocin. Can dislodge uric-acid stones, causing discomfort of the ureters. Safe for nursing mothers.

Skullcap *(Scutellaria spp.)*

Uses: Neurasthenia; depression with agitated states and oversensitivity to surroundings; feeling overstimulated. Pain with agitation and/or depression. Insomnia, fear, migraines, nervous headaches. Inability to concentrate due to a dull frontal headache or a headache located at the base of the brain. Helps control rage and anger, nervous heart disorders. Good for mentally overworked individuals. Relieves the nerve pain in herpes before eruptions occur. Calms delirium tremens. Calms agitation and irritation, as well as transitory pain, in cases of multiple sclerosis and neuralgia. Anti-inflammatory for nerve pain in general. Sciatica. Helpful in some cases of fibromyalgia.

Parts Used: Herb, recently dried

Constituents: Flavonoids, iridoids, volatile oil, tannins.

Dosage: Standard infusion, 2 to 6 ounces up to 3 times daily.

Notes: As mentioned above, skullcap is good for people who experience neurasthenia. This isn't as common a psycho-pathological diagnosis as it once was and is no longer even recognized by the American Psychiatric Association. Neurasthenia is a condition that includes anxiety, fatigue, headaches, aches and pains, and depression. Sounds like a common malady, doesn't it? It was once so commonly diagnosed in this country that it gained the nickname "Americanitis" in the mid 1800s. While I've no doubt scores of Americans are still suffering from this one, you'll have to visit Asia to gain your diagnosis. There, it's still recognized. I wonder if over there they call it "Asianitis"?

While any species of Scutellaria is good, the most impressive of the bunch is Scutellaria galericulata, according to herbalist Michael Moore.

Warnings: Occasionally, skullcap is sold in commerce blended with the herb germander. You want to make sure that what you purchase is skullcap only.

Spearmint (*Mentha spicata* or *viridis* LINN.)

Uses: A fantastic stomach aid in general. Nervous indigestion. Nausea after a headache. Kidney and intestinal ailments. Good for a mother during delivery, either before, after, or during childbirth. Safe for all ages.

Parts Used: Herb

Constituents: Volatile oil, menthol, menthone, d-limonene, neomenthol, tannins, traces of essential oil containing approximately 50% carvone.

Dosage: Standard infusion as needed.

Notes: Spearmint is a common herb to add to tea blends, especially in combination with medicinal herbs not known for their wonderful flavor. I like adding it to herbal teas for cold and flu care because the fragrance is uplifting and energetic, yet soothing. Kids love this one.

Warnings: None known.

Spikenard *(Aralia racemosa)*

Uses: Helpful in cases of chest colds, chronic laryngitis, bronchitis, pneumonia, or pharyngitis with lots of mucous. Acute cough with wheezing and dry mucous. A good overall influenza remedy. Also helpful for the elderly who have smoked for many years. Modulates blood sugar spikes, both high and low; good for type 2 diabetes, especially in its early stages. Good for people who dwell on past stresses. Delayed menses, especially as a result of a stressful month.

Parts Used: Root

Constituents: Choline, chlorogenic acid, ursolic acids, b-sitosterol, araloside, oleanic acid glycosides, several panaxosides.

Dosage: Strong decoction or cold infusion, 2 to 4 ounces up to 3 times daily.

Notes: When combined with squaw vine (Mitchella repens) and raspberry leaf teas, it's a good uterine tonic to be used in the last few weeks of pregnancy - under medical supervision, of course.

Warnings: None known.

Stinging Nettles (*Urtica dioica*)

Uses: Spring tonic. Nutrient-rich daily tea which helps rebuild and cleanse the body after a long winter. Supports the immune system, urinary tract, respiratory tract, circulation, nervous, digestive, and endocrine systems. Supportive in hay fever, allergies, and asthma. A good aid for chronic inflammation. Chronic cystorrhea. Excessive mucous discharge. Chronic respiratory, digestive, and urinary tract illnesses. Aids in cases of malnutrition, such as after a long illness or a major surgery. Anemia. Skin inflammation, as experienced in hives, eczema, chicken pox, and psoriasis. Hair loss. Arthritis, gout relief. Hypothyroid. Leg cramps. Premenstrual cramps. Profuse menstruation. Suppressed lactation. Low blood pressure. Male impotence. Good for individuals who are tired all the time with low energy.

Parts Used: Whole above-ground plant

Constituents: Chlorophyll; indoles such as histamine and serotonin; acetylcholine; flavonol glycosides; vitamin C and others; protein; dietary fiber; significant amounts of calcium, magnesium, potassium, silicic acid, and iron.

Dosage: Cold or standard infusion as needed. For the release of more mineral content, you may do a standard decoction or an overnight cold infusion.

Notes: As you can see, nettles are an herbal powerhouse! It's a nutritive herb, which means it's good to think of it as a food. Long-term use is not only safe but advised, especially when dealing with chronic illnesses.

Warnings: While this herb is safe for use during pregnancy, it should be consumed within reasonable levels. More is not better, so excessive doses are not recommended for pregnant women.

Stone Root *(Collinsonia canadensis)*

Uses: Good for treating stone and gravel in the gallbladder and urinary system, as it helps the body to pass stones. Also helps prevent new stones from forming. Strong diuretic herb. Hemorrhoids. Rheumatic inflammation. Laryngitis. Dysentery. Ulcers. Middle ear inflammation. Acute cystitis, urethritis, and vaginitis. Chronic cystitis and urethritis with dark or strained urination. Chronic vulvitis.

Parts Used: Root and herb

Constituents: Essential oil, tannins, saponins, alkaloids, resins, organic acid.

Dosage: Strong decoction, 8 to 10 ounces up to 3 times daily.

Notes: The root of the stone root looks — you guessed it — like a stone. It's about that hard, too, so cultivating it is no easy task.

Warnings: None known.

Strawberry *(Fragaria vesca, virginiana)*

Uses: Relieves nervousness in people and animals. As a mouth rinse for periodontal disease and loose teeth. Dry lungs. Diarrhea, dysentery. Irregular menses with excessive bleeding. Vaginal yeast infections. Use externally for eczema, psoriasis, and hives. Can be used as an eyewash for red, dry, irritated eyes.

Parts Used: Whole above-ground plant

Constituents: Tannins, antioxidant flavonoids, trace amounts of ascorbic acid and essential oil.

Dosage: Standard infusion as needed.

Notes: Strawberry is a member of the rose family, and it's full of tannins which give it its healing power. And you thought it was just for shortcake.

Warnings: None known.

T

Thyme *(Thymus vulgaris)*

Uses: Cold, flu, fevers. Also relieves coughs, whooping cough, bronchitis, pneumonia, and asthma. Loosens mucous in upper respiratory tract. Laryngitis, sore throat, tonsillitis. Indigestion, colic, diarrhea, flatulence relief. Good for urinary tract infections. Use externally for athlete's foot or ringworm.

Parts Used: Herb

Constituents: Volatile oils including thymol and smaller amounts of carvacrol; flavonoids, labiatic acid, caffeic acid, tannins.

Dosage: Standard infusion, 2 to 4 ounces up to 4 times daily.

Notes: Thyme grows very well in my garden. You can pretty much ignore it and it still grows just fine. In Medieval times, the thyme plant represented courage.   A courageous plant, indeed, that survives in my herb garden!

Warnings: Not for use in pregnancy, although it's still safe to cook with. Those who have duodenal ulcers or thyroid disease should not use thyme for medicinal purposes.

U

Uva Ursi *or* Manzanita (*Arctostaphylos uva ursi*)

Uses: A disinfecting herb that makes it a great choice for cystitis, nephritis, urethritis, and all types of urinary tract infections. Antilithitic for bladder and kidney stones. Clears cloudy urine. Incontinence. Discharges due to gonorrhea in women.

Parts Used: Leaves

Constituents: Hydroquinones; flavonoids; tannins; volatile oil; ursolic, malic, and gallic acids.

Dosage: Standard infusion, 3 to 4 ounces up to 3 times daily.

Notes: Uva ursi is closely related to cranberry. Like its cousin, it has a long history of use for urinary tract infections. Just don't serve it on Thanksgiving.

Warnings: Prolonged use may cause stomach irritations, so it should not be used for more than 3 or 4 days in a row. Not to be used during pregnancy. May turn urine temporarily green, but this is no cause for concern.

V

Valerian (*Valeriana spp.*)

Uses: A wonderful nerve tonic for emotional distress, hysteria, and restlessness. Heart palpitations due to nervousness. High blood pressure from stress. Effective as a heavy pain reliever. Also assists in cases of delirium tremens; insomnia; and neuralgia in convalescence. Helpful for poor cerebral circulation that causes nervous issues. Bouts of flatulence and depression after eating. Pain, intestinal cramps, menstrual cramps. Pain relief in shingles. Temporal, frontal headaches.

Parts Used: Whole plant or root

Constituents: Sesquiterpenes, monoterpenes, valepotriates, alkaloids, lignans, arginine, glutamine, tyrosine.

Dosage: Standard infusion, 4 to 6 ounces up to 2 times daily.

159

Notes: Valerian is easy to grow in the garden. While most commercially sold valerian is the dried root, the leaves work very well indeed. Biggest difference here: the root stinks to high heaven and, in my opinion, smells like cat pee. The leaves do not. The other advantage: When you dry and use the leaves for tea, you avoid what I refer to as "valerianism," which is an unpleasant and depressed feeling that can happen if you use the tea for more than a few weeks in a row.

Warnings: If you choose to use dried root for tea, it should be for short-term use only. Long-term use of more than a few weeks can result in mental agitation or depression. This does not seem to occur when using the dried above-ground plant.

W

Wahoo (*Euonymus atropurpureus*)

Uses: An excellent liver herb, it relieves congestion in the liver and aids in freeing the flow of the bile. Supports digestion. Used for treating jaundice. Gallbladder inflammation and pain with stones. Constipation with a poor appetite. Good for chronic anorexia nervosa paired with recurring viral infections or anorexia due to chemotherapy or other cancer therapies.

Parts Used: Root

Constituents: Cardenolides, alkaloids, sterols.

Dosage: Cold infusion, 1 to 2 ounces up to 2 times daily.

Notes: Did I add this one just because I like to say "wahoo"? Okay, maybe a little. Also known as "burningbush," you might just have one growing in your yard. It's a popular garden shrub that turns bright red in the fall and is a favorite in landscaping.

Warnings: Not to be used with cardiac glycosides or other cardioactive agents.

Wild Yam (*Dioscorea villosa*)

Uses: Relieves neuralgic and urinary tract pain. A general antispasmodic for gall bladder inflammation. Pain relief for renal and bladder colic. Colic, in general, for infants, children, and adults. A general antispasmodic for nausea and vomiting. Diarrhea and tenesmus. General relief of nervous system irritations. Inflamed uterus with cramping. Morning sickness. One of the best known herbal remedies for painful menses. Is sometimes used in cases of threatened miscarriage.

Parts Used: Root

Constituents: .5-1.2% diosgenin.

Dosage: Cold infusion, 2 to 4 ounces up to 4 times daily.

Notes: The wild yam is a vine with heart-shaped leaves and a white tuber that Native Americans used to rely on as a vegetable. It has been used as a natural birth control, but if you're really not planning on adding another family member, please do talk to a professional health care provider or a qualified herbalist before relying on it. I don't want to find out you had a surprise while taking wild yam and named the new baby "That Darned Kidman."

Warnings: None known.

Wild Cherry (*Prunus virginiana*)

Uses: Coughing, especially hot, dry, and frantic. Acute flu with coughing. Mild bronchitis; a good supportive aid for getting over bronchitis. Acute bronchial pneumonia. Acute gastritis with a cough. Spasmodic coughing in infants. A good aid for feverish viral infections that include shallow, rapid breathing and hot, dry membranes. Asthma, tuberculosis, pneumonia. Old coughs you can't seem to get rid of. Chronic gastritis with tenderness in the abdomen. Chronic diarrhea. Celiac and food allergies with irritation of the small intestine. Herpes, shingles. Fevers that have hung around awhile. Settles

163

down nervous irritability. Arthritis. Good choice for any age.

Parts Used: Summer or fall bark

Constituents: Cyanogenic glycosides, tannins, gallic acid, resin, hydrocyanic acid, benzaldehyde, eudesmic acid, p-coumaric acid, scopoletin, sugars.

Dosage: Cold infusion, 2 to 6 ounces up to 3 times daily.

Notes: Wild cherry is of great benefit to any home herbalist. The tea is delicious and indeed has a pleasing cherry flavor that kids will enjoy. Its ability to soothe the cough is widely recognized, and the tea brings the relief in a most delicious way.

Warnings: Not to be used during pregnancy. Not to be used over long periods of time due to the cyanogenic glycosides, which can be toxic in large amounts.

Willow (*Salix spp.*)

Uses: Contains salicin and is the natural source of aspirin, therefore making it a good natural alternative to aspirin. It has anti-inflammatory properties which make it a nice choice for relief of arthritis and joint pain, as well as general pain relief for things such as headaches in general, feverish headaches more specifically. Rheumatism. Acute cystitis or urethritis with aching, burning, scanty urination, inflamed urethral opening; analgesic. Hay fever relief. Good as an astringent gargle.

Parts Used: Bark

Constituents: Salicin, salicylic acids, tannins, catechin, p-coumaric acid, flavonoids.

Dosage: Strong decoction, 2 to 4 ounces up to 4 times daily.

Notes: If you have willow trees growing in your yard or you plan to harvest your own bark, please be sure to choose bark from a tree that is not sprayed or treated in any way. I prefer collecting the bark from the twigs of spring growth. Never, ever strip the bark all the way around any tree trunk in a circle.

That will certainly kill the tree.

Warnings: Not for use by those with allergies to aspirin or salicylates.

Wild Ginger (*Asarum caudatum*)

Uses: Beginning of a head cold with a dry fever; viral infections. Chronic cough. Flatulent colic. Indigestion. Dry, hot skin. Pneumonia paired with overexhaustion. Measles, chicken pox, scarlet fever, smallpox, typhoid fever. Fever in infants, children, or adults with suppressed sweating. Warms up a cold body and keeps it warm. Delayed menses, especially when due to a recent viral infection or from exposure to cold weather; or when menses is suppressed even after passing a clot. Postpartum depression. Slight muscarinic effect.

Parts Used: Leaves

Dosage: Standard infusion, 2 to 4 ounces up to 2 times daily.

Notes: I grow wild ginger in the garden, and not just for its medicinal properties. The leaves are a gorgeous iridescent green in the sunlight, and the flowers are quite unusual, although you have to stand on your head to see them. They hang down from the plant and hide under the leaves, but definitely worth the head rush.

Warnings: Not for use during pregnancy. Drinking a cup or more at once can cause nausea, even vomiting. Keep to small doses.

Wintergreen (*Gaultheria procumbens*)

Uses: A pain reducer and anti-inflammatory offering relief to numerous aches and pains. Good for arthritis and swollen joints. Diuretic. Chronic cystitis, urethritis with prostatitis. Acute painful urination with back pain, difficulty in urinating. Hemorrhoids of the painful, extruding type. General headache relief for children.

Parts Used: Leaves, recently dried or fresh

Constituents: Arbutin, caffeic acid, ericolin, ferulic acid, gaultherase, gaultheric acid, gaultherin, primverose, tannins, vanillic acid,

Dosage: Standard infusion, 2 to 4 ounces as needed.

Notes: The leaves of the wintergreen should be stored in a container with a tight-fitting lid and away from the light. My own personal stash seems to be good for about a year if I've collected and dried it myself. If purchased in commerce, it may already be old by the time you get it, so give it a whiff if you can. Fresh wintergreen has a clean, strong smell. A pleasant tasting tea.

Warnings: None known.

Y

Yarrow (*Achillea millefolium*)

Uses: Cold, flu relief. Drink the tea cold to relieve chills associated with cold and flu. Also breaks a fever. Aids in respiratory infections. Indigestion, nausea. Stops a bloody nose. If used topically, it's good for cuts and abrasions. General hemorrhage, stops passive internal bleeding. Used for the coughing up or spitting of blood. Heavy menses, especially when bright red blood present, such as with fibroids; drink cold in this case. Also helps in cases of suppressed menses. Diarrhea relief. Varicose veins and hemorrhoids. Appetite stimulant. Good to cleanse liver after a drinking binge, after eating lots of low quality foods, or after a bad case of diarrhea such as one that may occur from traveling overseas.

Parts Used: Whole flowering herb

Constituents: Volatile oils, sesquiterpene lactones, tannins, flavonoids, alkaloids, phenolic acids.

Dosage: Standard infusion, 2 to 4 ounces up to 3 times daily.

Notes: Yarrow tastes minty but is a little on the weird side. Sort of like minty dirt. But it's so useful that I'm never without it.

Warnings: Yarrow is not recommended for children with a history of elevated temperatures and seizures. Otherwise safe for children.

Yellow Dock (*Rumex crispus*)

Uses: This blood purifier strengthens a weak colon when singular red eruptions on the buttocks and shoulders are present. Chronic constipation with singular red eruptions on the face, back, neck, or buttocks. Indigestion with liver congestion. Diarrhea (especially in the morning), dysentery, colitis. Speeds slow digestion. Acne with just a few large eruptions on face, neck, or buttocks. Eczema with boils. Chronic psoriasis brought on by irritable bowel syndrome (IBS) or colitis. Skin eruptions due to menstrual cycle.

Anemia due to menstrual issues. Suppressed menses. Rheumatism. Ulcers.

Parts Used: Root; sometimes leaves

Constituents: Anthraquinone glycosides, tannins, oxalates.

Dosage: Simple infusion, 2 to 4 ounces up to 3 times daily.

Notes: This is a good herb for constipation because it's gentle and, when used properly, won't make you crampy. Start with a small amount of tea and work your way up. If you do start to feel crampy, you've taken too much, so be conservative until you know what to expect from it.

Warnings: Use with caution if kidney stones present.

Yerba Mansa (*Anemopsis californica*)

Uses: Relieves subacute head colds with thick mucous. Acute or chronic pharyngitis. Acute or chronic sinusitis with inflammation, stuffy nose and congested head with a frontal headache. Chronic bronchitis. Chronic tonsillitis. Asthma with moist cough. Good for mouth, gum, and throat sores. Acute cystitis or urethritis with mucous in urine. Diarrhea recuperation or recuperating after an intestinal infection. Painful extruding hemorrhoids. Nausea after eating. Ulcers with vomiting. Vomiting in general. Appendicitis. A diuretic and anti-inflammatory for arthritis. Infant teething with cold sores (used topically). Rheumatoid arthritis relief; its anti-inflammatory properties and diuretic effect removes uric acid. Pre-eclampsia, vaginitis. Antibacterial, antifungal. Apply topically for athlete's foot.

Parts Used: Root and/or herb

Constituents: Methyl eugenol and related compounds, estragole, thymol methyl ether, linalool, p-cymene, asarinin, aromatics.

Dosage: When preparing the root, use a cold or standard infusion. 2 to 4 ounces up to 5 times daily. For the herb, use a cold or standard infusion as needed.

Notes: Yerba mansa is becoming more and more rare in the wild and is recognized as a plant at risk by the United Plant Savers (www.unitedplantsavers.org), so if you plan to pick your own, consider growing it yourself if you're in USDA Zones 8 or 9. Plants can be purchased from nurseries in those areas. Instead of taking more from an already fragile environment, you can help propagate a useful herb!

Warnings: None known.

Yerba Mate (*Ilex paraguariensis*)

Uses: A nice remedy for headaches, hangovers, etc. Caffeinated; a good substitute for coffee for those who have gastritis or colitis, it wakes you up without a shaky feeling. Refreshes, invigorates. Good for mental alertness.

Parts Used: Leaves

Constituents: Tannins, antioxidants, polyphenols, amino acids, saponins, vitamins, flavonoids.

Dosage: Standard infusion as needed.

Notes: This is one of my favorite teas, and I probably drink a cup every day. Ever since I read an Argentinean novel in which the starving artists would do just about anything to get their mate, I have been enamored with it. Mate gourds and metal straws are the proper tools for drinking the tea, but you can also make a standard infusion and enjoy it that way. Very similar in taste to green tea, it's a great pick-me-up, and I've noticed it improves concentration and opens the mind. It's extremely healthy and contains a whopping 196 active compounds!

Warnings: Not for use by those who cannot have caffeine.

Clark's Rule

When giving infants and children herbs that are deemed safe for them, it's important to make sure you've got the dosage correct. Clark's Rule is a standard that many herbalists use to determine the correct amount of herb for infants and young children.

Here's what you do: Take the weight of the child in pounds and divide that weight by 150. This will give an approximate fraction of the adult dosage you'll use. For instance, a child that weighs 50 pounds will receive ⅓ the adult dose since $50/150 = ⅓$.

Herbal Shopping Guide

Blessed Herbs - A supplier that caters to herbalists, retail stores, etc. Dried herbs, beeswax, extracts, and more.
www.blessedherbs.com

Flack Family Farm - Located in Vermont, they sell certified organic products, including fresh and dried herbs.
www.flackfamilyfarm.com/medherbs.html

Friends of the Trees - A good resource for herb infused oils, either in small quantities or bulk. Lots of other fun things happening on this site. Books, a plethora of news articles and resources, and more.
www.friendsofthetrees.net/index.htm

Frontier Natural Products Co-op - My local health food store carries dried herbs from Frontier, and I've had nothing but good product from them. Love the henna!
www.frontiercoop.com

Healing Spirits Herb Farm - Located in western New York, this farm sells a large variety of items, including dried and fresh herbs and roots, tinctures, extracts, and teas. A beautiful site and a lovely selection.

www.healingspiritsherbfarm.com/store/258

Heartsong Farm - A family farm that grows organic and ethically harvested wild herbs. They like to focus on providing optimal medicinal quality herbs.

www.herbsandapples.com

Horizon Herbs - Dried herbs, herbal extracts, live plants; even buy your own vegetable seeds or medicinal plant seeds and grow your own from scratch.

www.horizonherbs.com

Mountain Rose Herbs - An online Mecca of all things herbal. The site is seemingly endless and fun to browse through.

www.mountainroseherbs.com

Pacific Botanicals - A large all-organic herb farm in Oregon. They have an impressive list of goods, including fresh and dried herbs, organic seeds, even sea vegetables.

www.pacificbotanicals.com

Starwest Botanicals - Another great online herb store that'll blow your mind. A huge selection of just about everything.
www.starwest-botanicals.com

Taos Herb Co. - Located in one of the coolest cities in the country, Taos Herb Co. offers essential oils, dried herbs, a wide selection of sage, and all sorts of fun gift items such as soapstone diffusers.
www.taosherb.com

The Herbalist - Bulk dried organic herbs, organic essential oils at a fair price, flower essences, etc.
www.theherbalist.com

Zack Woods Herbs - Bulk dried herbs, fresh herbs and roots, even whole plants! It's a family farm that supplies high quality organic herbs. Can't beat that!
www.zackwoodsherbs.com

180

Bibliography

Balch, Phyllis A., CNC. Prescription for Herbal Healing. New York, NY: Avery, 2002.

Hoffmann, David, FNIMH, AHG. Medical Herbalism: The Science and Practice of Herbal Medicine. Rochester, VT: Healing Arts Press, 2003.

Hoffmann, David, FNIMH, AHG. The Herbal Handbook: A User's Guide to Medical Herbalism. Rochester, VT: Healing Arts Press, 1998.

Jones, Feather. Medicinal Herb Handbook: An Herbal Application Guide for Novice and Clinician through Simplified Herbal Remedy Descriptions. Twin Lakes, WI: Lotus Press, 1999.

Moore, Michael. Los Remedios: Traditional Herbal Remedies of the Southwest. Santa Fe, NM: Museum of New Mexico Press, 1990.

Moore, Michael. Medicinal Plants of the Desert and Canyon West. Santa Fe, NM: Museum of New Mexico Press, 1989.

Smith, Ed. Therapeutic Herb Manual: A Guide to the Safe and Effective Use of Liquid Herbal Extracts. Williams, OR: Ed Smith, 2008.

Tilgner, Sharol Marie N.D. Herbal Medicine from the Heart of the Earth. Pleasant Hill, OR: Wise Acres, LLC, 2009.

Wood, Matthew. The Earthwise Herbal: A Complete Guide to Old World Medicinal Plants. Berkeley, CA: North Atlantic Books, 2008.

Wood, Matthew. The Earthwise Herbal: A Complete Guide to New World Medicinal Plants. Berkeley, CA: North Atlantic Books, 2009.

Other Books by Diane Kidman

Herbs Gone Wild! Ancient Remedies Turned Loose

Beauty Gone Wild! Herbal Recipes for Gorgeous Skin & Hair

Hair Gone Wild! Recipes & Remedies for Natural Tresses

Acknowledgements

Thanks to my husband and son who both tolerated my papers and books spread all over the living room, dining room, and various furniture surfaces while this compilation went from a complete mess of scrap paper and notes to a cohesive volume. Your support and love keep me going! In fact, the enthusiasm of my entire extended family makes me feel like I'm a giggly five-year-old again. To my dogs and birds, you could tune the noise level down a bit during writing hours, but your warm fur and feathers are much appreciated at the end of a long day.